THE
ORIGINS
OF YOU

THE ORIGINS OF YOU

How Breaking Family Patterns
Can Liberate the Way
We Live and Love

VIENNA PHARAON

LICENSED MARRIAGE AND FAMILY THERAPIST

G. P. PUTNAM'S SONS
NEW YORK

PUTNAM
— EST. 1838 —

G. P. PUTNAM'S SONS
Publishers Since 1838
An imprint of Penguin Random House LLC
penguinrandomhouse.com

Library of Congress Cataloging-in-Publication Data

Names: Pharaon, Vienna, author.
Title: The origins of you: how breaking family patterns can liberate the way we live and love / Vienna Pharaon, licensed marriage and family therapist.
Description: New York: G. P. Putnam's Sons, 2023. |
Includes bibliographical references and index.
Identifiers: LCCN 2022050393 (print) | LCCN 2022050394 (ebook) |
ISBN 9780593539910 (hardcover) | ISBN 9780593539927 (ebook)
Subjects: LCSH: Adult children of dysfunctional families—Mental health—Popular works. |
Adult children of dysfunctional families—Rehabilitation—Popular works. |
Adult children of dysfunctional families—Case studies. |
Families—Psychological aspects—Popular works.
Classification: LCC RC455.4.F3 P43 2023 (print) | LCC RC455.4.F3 (ebook) |
DDC 362.2085—dc23/eng/20221021
LC record available at https://lccn.loc.gov/2022050393
LC ebook record available at https://lccn.loc.gov/2022050394

Printed in the United States of America
1st Printing

All names and identifying characteristics of the author's clients have been changed to protect the individuals' privacy.

*To my soul helpers
Connor, Code, and Bronx.
You are everything good in this world.*

CONTENTS

Author's Note   ix

Introduction: My Family of Origin and Yours   1

PART I
OUR ROOTS

1. Your Past Is Your Present   17

2. Naming Your Wound   31

PART II
OUR WOUNDS AND THEIR ORIGINS

3. I Want to Feel Worthy   57

4. I Want to Belong   85

5. I Want to Be Prioritized   109

6. I Want to Trust   135

7. I Want to Feel Safe   157

CONTENTS

PART III
CHANGING YOUR RELATIONSHIP BEHAVIORS

8. Conflict   185

9. Communication   210

10. Boundaries   236

PART IV
YOUR RECLAMATION

11. Making It Stick   255

Conclusion   269

Acknowledgments   273

Notes   277

Index   283

AUTHOR'S NOTE

I wouldn't have been able to write this book without the great honor of intimately working alongside so many incredible humans who chose to bravely share their stories with me. I have made it a priority to disguise all identities and recognizable details of my clients. In a few cases, I've combined aspects of multiple clients and attributed them to one. All stories are true in spirit, and I've made sure that any changes made still honor the individual's story.

Also, a note that abuse, suicide, and severe mental health challenges are topics in chapter 7, "I Want to Feel Safe." Please be mindful as you read.

Finally, as much as I hope you will find parts of yourself throughout, this book by necessity does not cover everything. Change is different and challenging for everyone, and the revelations you come into contact with here may feel destabilizing at times or introduce new dynamics with your family. Working with a therapist as you navigate the relational healing you're seeking may be supportive. This is especially true for those working to heal their trauma, which often requires a more involved approach. If you've experienced trauma or complex trauma, you will likely benefit from working with a trauma-informed clinician.

THE ORIGINS OF YOU

INTRODUCTION: MY FAMILY OF ORIGIN AND YOURS

I was just five years old when a rupture in my family left me with a wound that would dictate the course of my relationships for years to come.

For a long time I refused to acknowledge the effect my past had had on, well, *everything* else in my life. In fact, I might never have fully understood the importance of these early events without an education in psychology, a working knowledge of the lingering effects of trauma, and a deep curiosity around relationships. It has taken me years of hard work to see the impact of what happened long ago and to actively take control of who I want to be in relationships, valuable lessons I've learned that I will share with you in this book. But I'm getting ahead of myself. Let's start at the beginning.

Let's start with my origins.

It was a beautiful sunny day in the summer of 1991. I was trying to make a flimsy gold bangle into a trendy hoop earring—five going on fifteen, as they say—when I heard my father's raised voice from behind the closed bedroom door. My father's anger was always scary to me. He was the kind of man who often dominated situations he was in, and the power and control he exuded felt threatening and manipulative. My joy in my cool jewelry project immediately vanished.

1

"If you leave, don't come back," he shouted at my mother.

The words pierced me. I'd never heard such rage targeted at someone I loved, at someone he was supposed to love: *If you leave, don't come back.*

Within minutes my mom was barreling upstairs, urging me to pack a bag. There wasn't much time for my system to process what was happening. All I knew was that we were leaving.

We picked up my maternal grandmother and went to the Jersey Shore, where I am sure I played in the waves, built castles in the sand, and probably convinced my mom to stop for ice cream on the way home. It hadn't yet struck me that "home" this time might mean somewhere else. Dropping off my grandmother wouldn't be just another stop. It was the destination.

When we got to my grandma's house, we settled in, unwinding after a day in the sun. It wasn't long before the phone started to ring. Although there was no caller ID at the time, it was obvious who was on the other end of the line. My father immediately demanded to speak to my mom, but my grandma knew better than to pass her the phone. Within minutes, we were all running over to the neighbor's house. No time to process. Just time to run.

About ten minutes later my father and his brother, my uncle, pulled into my grandma's driveway. We watched from afar as they banged on the front door, circled the house, and tried to catch a glimpse of any movement inside. My mom's parked car was a clear giveaway that we couldn't be far. I remember ever so carefully peeking my head above the windowsill to see what was going on just a house away. My dad and uncle were just small figures in the distance, but I could still see their rage.

I wanted to call out to my dad, but I was also frightened. I was hiding with my mom, feeling terrified and unsafe, while simultaneously thinking to myself, *I'm right here, Dad.*

Minutes later, the police pulled into my grandmother's driveway.

I could hear the fear in my mom's voice as she demanded I hide in the closet with her. *This is really happening.* I was instructed to not make a peep. Then came the knock, which pierced in a familiar way. The neighbor opened the door to two angry men and a couple of police officers. The questions came from the officers while accusations came from my father and uncle. They knew we were inside, but there was no invitation to enter.

I could hear the rage escalating. *There must be something I can do to fix this,* I prayed. *How do I make this stop? I just want them both to be okay.*

Yet there was no way to make both of my parents happy. There was no way to choose them both. There was no way to honor one without hurting or disappointing the other, or so I believed. There was no way to stop the fight.

Throughout the incident, we remained, my mom and me, stock-still, hand in hand, in the closet.

And though I didn't then have the language to describe it, it was then—at that moment—my own safety wound was born. I had no idea, at the time, just how long I would remain trapped in that moment.

Even though my parents tried their best, they couldn't protect me or shield me from their rage. My physical safety was never threatened, but the system I called my family was crashing and burning. The chaos became the status quo. I saw two adults come face-to-face with threats, exhibiting manipulation, paranoia, emotional flooding, abuse, control, and fear. As much as they tried to hide it from me, I saw it, I felt it, and I experienced it alongside them. My world had suddenly, dramatically, become unsafe. The two people whom I'd trusted to be my protectors were so busy fighting each other they for a time lost sight of me.

I realized I had to create my own safety.

I took on the role of peacekeeper in an attempt to put out the fire and to keep the family functioning. It was quite the role for a five-year-old. Unaware that it wasn't my responsibility, I gave it everything I had. I became a phenomenal actress. I had determined that my not being okay at all times was too much for my parents to face, so I'd say, "I'm fine," with the sole intention of not adding to their burden. And in an effort to always please them and tell them what I believed they needed to hear, I never shared my preferences, only validated theirs. I became a child with no needs of her own, exceptional at anything I put my mind to, always helping to lessen the burden or distract them from what was happening.

My safety wound—more about this in the pages that follow—remained unaddressed and, repeatedly reinjured, continued to unconsciously direct my life. I was always on the alert, always ready to put out the next potential fire, whether the kindling and match came from my parents, my friends, or eventually my own partners. But the long-term effects of taking on this inappropriate peacekeeper role and of mistakenly putting all my efforts into making everything okay would take years to unpack. I learned to shapeshift, shrink, minimize, maximize, and distort myself and my experiences all in the name of pleasing—a habit I would later need to work tirelessly at overthrowing if I wanted to have authentic relationships.

And I became so skilled at making sure that what happened to my parents didn't happen to me that I wound up re-creating everything I was fearful of. My fear of being controlled, as my father had controlled my mother, made me controlling myself. My people-pleasing and need to be worthy made me invulnerable and inauthentic, blocking genuine connections. And my cool-girl, on-top-of-everything persona made it impossible for me to reveal how I really felt or to ask for any of my needs to be met. I was stuck in my personal and professional relationships, re-creating the very patterns I'd sworn to never repeat.

When I first started therapy, I didn't see any of this. I was convinced that the issue I needed to work on was "improving communication and conflict in my relationships." I found myself inexplicably at odds with people in all aspects of my life—friends, colleagues, and especially people I dated—but somehow I never traced these different frustrations and struggles back to this inciting incident in my childhood. *I survived that,* I told myself. *I kept the peace.*

But deep down I knew better. The underlying problem (what all that conflict was *really* about) went back to that terror-filled day. It went back to my family of origin and my resulting safety wound. And it was only then—when I began to explore myself through the lens of my family of origin—that I finally began to become unstuck.

Suddenly, when viewed through this new perspective, my way of being and existing started to make sense. I saw how a finite experience that happened decades ago had had an enduring effect on me. I had attempted to ignore the original wound that had shattered my sense of safety and to sidestep the resulting pain—becoming the one who tried to fly under the radar in an effort to avoid adding any additional stress to my family, and in every subsequent relationship.

Spoiler alert: Trying not to add stress to others only created stress and more pain for myself. White-knuckling my way through conflict without properly acknowledging the origin of it didn't work in my own relationships as an adult. Neither did my other defense mechanism—the cool-girl, above-it-all persona. My attempts to avoid pain and keep myself "safe" were having the exact opposite effect. By hiding how *I really felt,* by failing to embrace my needs or express myself, I was tamping down conflict only for it to reemerge in other places. And in hiding from my pain and wound—in not even seeing that there *was* something that needed my attention—I denied my own healing.

The good news—which I learned from hard work, both on myself and with my hundreds of clients over fifteen years as a marriage and family therapist—is that it doesn't have to be this way. Just because we have wounds from our childhoods doesn't mean we are doomed to repeat those patterns. If we pause to understand where these wounds come from (our origin stories) and take the time to make different choices, we can access powerful healing. In fact, our origin stories can be the road map to our healing, once we are willing to really look.

I've worked with clients in more than 20,000 hours of therapy over my career. I also run an Instagram community of over 600,000 individuals with whom I'm in conversation daily. In this book I share my own stories and the stories of many others I've worked with. Their names are changed and many of the details of their lives are altered to protect their identity, but their stories are offered with the aim of reflecting something back to you, with the aim of helping you truly see yourself and others. I want to help you explore your own origin stories, naming your wounds, making the connection between those wounds and your unhealthy behaviors, and ultimately learning how to create and maintain healthy relationships in your life right now.

This book will teach you how to look beyond what we in the therapy world call the *presenting problem,* the problem that you come to therapy to resolve. It will ask you to explore and connect with the *origins* of your beliefs, behaviors, and patterns, and the way your family of origin contributed to them. Most of the damaging and frustrating patterns we find ourselves in originate with wounds we sustained in childhood. Understanding your *origin wound* and the long-standing destructive patterns it leads to, will go a long way to addressing conflicts and behaviors that trouble you today.

The work begins with our family of origin. This is where the foundation of how we relate to others, ourselves, and the world around us begins to take shape. Your early relationships—the presence of them, the absence, the negligence, the hypervigilance—all have an impact on how you view just about everything in your life today. Your family of origin may have been consistently functional, sometimes functional, or rarely functional. Whatever the degree, it wasn't perfect. You craved things from them that they couldn't or didn't give to you, you needed protection from things they didn't (or did) see, and you wanted permission to feel and experience things they withheld as threatening to their way of feeling and experiencing.

The majority of the relationship difficulties that individuals or couples come to me with are due to lingering and unresolved pain and trauma from past relationships, especially within their family of origin. It's why I call what I do with my clients *origin healing work*.

Origin healing work is an integration of family systems work and psychodynamic theory. It's based on Integrative Systemic Therapy, which was the approach I learned when I trained to be a marriage and family therapist at Northwestern University. We look for how our present-day behavior connects to the family systems in which we grew up, and to see the issues a person is struggling with within the context of a much larger system around them.

When you don't do this work, as we'll learn in part 1, your pain and trauma tend to go unresolved. It doesn't matter how much you try to avoid that painful past: how far away you physically move ("the geographical cure," as psychologist Dr. Froma Walsh calls it) or whether you fully cut yourself off from a harmful family member. There is an internal resolution that must happen if you're going to heal, and that internal resolution requires an understanding and awareness of the origin wounds that have a tight grip on you.

I have yet to meet a person who doesn't have some kind of origin wound. In this book, we'll explore five that are common. In fact, you might recognize more than one in yourself. Maybe you struggled to feel worthy of love growing up. Maybe you always felt like you didn't belong. Maybe you questioned whether you were important enough to be a priority. Maybe you struggled to trust those closest to you, or maybe you didn't feel physically or emotionally safe.

Naming your origin wounds is the first step toward your healing. In each of the chapters in part 2, we will explore a specific wound's origins and the destructive ways you learned to cope with it, and then read some healing stories. I will then lead you through your own Origin Healing Practice, in which you'll work through for yourself a four-step process that includes the naming of the wound, its witnessing, grieving alongside of it (yup, we're going to do some feeling in these pages), and then pivoting, making the long-lasting changes so that you don't keep repeating the patterns you've been trying to break in your adult relationships. If you're ready to stop replaying your destructive dynamics with the important people in your life, you're going to want to pay attention to this healing work. And no, you can't skip over your pain. No matter how much you bargain with it, you can't avoid your origin wound and forge a new way forward. As the saying goes, the only way out is through. I'm here to walk alongside you on your path through.

Once you have a more thorough understanding of your origin wound, you'll be ready to see how those wounds and the patterns you learned in your family system more generally influence your relationship behaviors today. In part 3, we'll look specifically at how you learned to communicate and to navigate conflict, and what you learned (or didn't learn) about boundaries. As we learn more about your past patterns, I'll help you shift the way you communicate, fight, and set or lift boundaries to healthier ways of engagement and a more authentic way of being.

When you notice yourself becoming reactive or falling into a destructive pattern, you're going to get into the habit of asking yourself certain questions so you can process what's happening in a different manner than you normally do. It's not good enough to just know why you choose the same types of partners over and over again, and it's not good enough to know why you react the way you do. Origin healing work is also about finding a path forward where you can live out what you *know* and reclaim what has been taken with compassion, understanding, and empathy for yourself and often for others. We're going to focus on healing the past, but we're also going to take steps that disrupt and change the programming and conditioning that has kept you stuck in the present.

Throughout, there will be plenty of prompts, exercises, and guided meditations so that you can do the work as we go. You will start the process of freeing yourself from unwanted patterns and behaviors that sabotage your relationships and your life. You will take specific steps to get on the road to healing and self-discovery.

Let me be very clear here. This work is *not* about throwing parents, caretakers, or any of the adults who served as parental figures for you under the bus. (A note: Throughout this book, I mostly use the words *parents, caretakers,* or *adults,* but whenever you see those words, please recognize that they are interchangeable with any and all parental figures you had growing up.) In fact, when I work with clients, I explicitly don't point a finger or place blame. This work requires context, and if we can access them, grace and compassion. We ought to remember that our caregivers, too, have a rich history made up of flawed family systems and origin stories that laid the bricks to their way of being.

And though the point of the exploration is not to bash others, it also isn't about excusing harmful behavior. We explore to acknowledge and name our experiences without minimizing or invalidating them. Our families likely did the best with what they knew, but they still might have fallen short. Explaining away the harmful experiences doesn't change the work you need to do.

Your stories are also going to be different from mine and different from your neighbors'. Maybe you've faced many more traumatic events than most of the people you know, or maybe you feel grateful that your story isn't so bad. Wherever you believe you land on the spectrum, your story requires your gentle and deliberate attention.

Your work is to name, acknowledge, feel, and recognize the impact that your family of origin had on you—and to use that awareness and understanding as a guiding light to create healthy, lasting change for yourself. You will not arrive and be done one day. You will continue learning more about yourself, your partner, and your family. You will find reactivity in new places no matter your age. You will notice areas of grief that are still calling for your attention. And you will likely meet your hurt inner child time and time again, who will crave for your acknowledgment, your witnessing, your grief, and your presence.

Origin healing work has been both the path forward for me personally and the work that I do day in and day out with my clients. It creates an opportunity for change (long-lasting, integrated change), gets you unstuck, and offers a reclamation of beliefs and a remembering of what was true before the unintegrated pain and trauma of your family got passed to you.

I don't believe that there is only one path forward. I believe there are as many paths forward as there are humans walking this earth. But what I do know to be true is that when I started to explore my origin stories through the lens of my family system, my way of being and existing started to make sense, and healing became an offering I could accept.

Instead of choosing the same types of partners who would re-create my childhood wounding, I was able to choose a partner who was equally dedicated to rolling up his sleeves and meeting me in the hard work. The narrative I held around romantic relationships began to soften.

- Instead of needing to be fine all the time, I was able to show vulnerability to others—and figure out who in my life was deserving of seeing my true, vulnerable self.

- Instead of needing to be a peacekeeper and prioritize pleasing others, I learned to honor myself—even if it meant that I'd disappoint another.

- Instead of trying to get others to change, to take a different path, or to see the suffering they were living in, I acknowledged who they were—and I changed the way I related to their *not* changing.

- And instead of needing to be in control, I learned to trust that someone could lead me without taking advantage of me.

Our origin stories carry beautiful complexity and heartbreaking pain. My parents' separation became official in November of 1991, and my mother and I moved out in May of 1992. This began a nine-year process of divorce, the longest in the history of New Jersey at the time. There was a lot of fear and a lot of grief I had to process, even though their relationship shifted significantly and they're friendly today. I've spent years packing and unpacking the messages I received during that time. Many of the skills I use today as a therapist can be traced directly back to my years-long role pacifying and mediating

THE ORIGINS OF YOU

between my parents. As my dear friend and colleague Dr. Alexandra Solomon says, "Our wounds and our gifts are next-door neighbors." What a beautiful reminder that some of our greatest gifts do emerge from the pain we've endured.

Yet there is a happy ending. Having an intimate relationship with your origin stories is not just practice in getting to know oneself, getting to know one's family, or rehashing the past. An intimate relationship with them is an opportunity for healing—for you, for those who came before you, and for those who come after. As family therapist and author Terry Real says, "Family dysfunction rolls down from generation to generation, like a fire in the woods, taking down everything in its path until one person in one generation has the courage to turn and face the flames. That person brings peace to their ancestors and spares the children that follow." Will you face the flames?

It doesn't matter whether you've been in therapy for decades or whether therapy isn't for you. It doesn't matter if you've explored family systems work before or this is the first time you're considering it. It doesn't matter if you have loads of memories from childhood or struggle to remember anything at all. Sometimes the explicit memory goes away because the pain was so big, but you're still able to feel. What matters is your openness, your willingness to explore, to feel, and to see what might be hard to see, accept, or acknowledge. What matters is that you take good care of yourself as you move through this book, staying connected to whether you need to keep pushing through or pause for a moment.

How you use this book is up to you. There is no right or wrong way. You might choose to work through these chapters with your own therapist. You might choose to read it on your own in a deeply intimate way and reflect about what comes up. Or you might choose to read it with a partner, a family member, or a friend, and use it as a way to begin conversations.

Whatever path is for you, you are here because you are seeking something. You are here because you carry with you something that needs your attention. You are here because you are tired of the weight that you hold, the draining patterns you find yourself in, and the exhaustion of your very well-intentioned desire for change continually falling short. I see you, I hear you, I've been there before, and I'm thrilled to walk alongside you as you do this hard work.

To explore your origin stories is a courageous and remarkable step on your healing journey. Let's begin.

PART I

OUR ROOTS

1

YOUR PAST IS YOUR PRESENT

There wasn't much information on the intake form that was sent in. Just her name, age, and a small blurb about what she would like to work on.

Natasha Harris, 38

I need to figure out whether my partner is someone I can spend my life with. I've had concerns for a long time, but I feel like I can't look the other way anymore. Can you help?!

Natasha was new to therapy. Her friends finally convinced her to go talk to someone—me—and she was both nervous and excited for our first session.

"I so need this," she said. "Thank you for making room in your schedule to see me. I've been delaying this for a long time, and I know I can't anymore. Plus, my friends are so over me complaining to them." She laughed nervously.

I smiled.

"I guess it does get old when you hear the same old story over and over again. They've been hearing it since they've known me."

"How long have they known you?" I asked.

"Oh, we're childhood friends. We go way back. They've been my girls for thirty-plus years."

The complaints her friends were tired of hearing were not unique to this current partner. These complaints were the same she'd had about almost every partner since she began seriously dating.

"Can you tell me what it is they've been hearing from you?" I asked.

"Well, I guess I tell them it's more of a feeling, a sense that something's off. They tell me that I'm just *looking* for something to be wrong, you know? Like I'm just trying to sabotage a good thing. I don't know. I guess I *do* push away people who are good for me. That's what everyone says, so maybe it's true."

I could see Natasha in her head already. The words and messages from others had clearly infiltrated her narratives about herself. It was hard for her to know what *she* felt, to acknowledge what *she* knew, and to get clear on what was true for *her*.

"It sounds like your friends have a lot of thoughts about how you show up in relationships. But I'm curious to know what it is *you* know to be true of your partner and your relationship?"

"Okay, sure. Clyde is a great man. He's smart, attractive, interesting, successful, and so kind and thoughtful. When you look at Clyde, there isn't anything you can spot that's wrong with him. Everyone thinks he's a catch, and that I've finally met my match."

I interrupted her. "Do *you* think Clyde is a catch?" I was trying to move her back to her experience of him.

"I do. He's a wonderful partner to me. He's a great man and I really don't have any complaints of him. I just think something is off or that something *will* be off. Maybe I'm missing something, you know? Like, what if the other shoe drops at some point?"

"Has the other shoe dropped in other relationships?"

My sudden departure from Clyde seemed to surprise her.

"I don't think so, no," she responded.

"Did the other shoe drop in your family ever?" I continued.

She paused, looking at me with a puzzled expression. "I really don't think this is related to my family. Why do therapists always like to bring it back to that? Honestly, my childhood was pretty great. I don't think you're going to find much there. I'd rather just figure out what's going on with Clyde."

It's in moments like these that I get a good internal (loving!) chuckle and think about Brené Brown from her TEDx talk "The Power of Vulnerability," where she famously tried to set a boundary with her therapist in their first session: "no family stuff, no childhood shit, I just need some strategies."

Spoiler alert: That approach didn't work for Brené, and it won't work for you, either. Because whether you want to admit it or not, the "family stuff" and "childhood shit" are at the root of, well, *everything*.

I know, I know, this may not be what you wanted to hear. You may even be adamant that the stuff that happened so long ago doesn't affect you at all today. You've grown and evolved, right? Maybe you've even forgiven. It's hard to believe that things from decades ago are still running the show and ruling your life.

But here's the thing I know for sure: your past creates patterns that affect your life today.

So even if you have evolved, even if you've grown in significant ways, even if you're not the same person you used to be . . . you're still a link in a multigenerational chain. And whether you're aware of it, that larger family system is guiding parts of your life in ways large and small. More likely than not, your past is running the show—*your show*—and if you're not conscious of it, you are likely suffering from it.

The past is persistent, my friend. The more you turn away from it, the more it follows you and asks for your attention. Ever wonder why you fight about the same things, over and over again? Ever wonder why you keep choosing the same types of partners? Ever wonder why you react the same way, no matter how hard you try to change it? Or why your inner critic repeats the same unkind things to you? That's your past asking for attention. That "childhood shit" directs your life in some way today that you would benefit from knowing about.

By choosing not to spend time on her childhood, Natasha has actually revealed a lot. Within a split second I know that it's going to take a little work before she and I are co-explorers on this journey. She's not there yet, and that's okay. But what's so exciting is that this journey into her family's story will inevitably uncover important links between her past and her present. She'll see connections between her family of origin and the questions swirling around her life today. If she keeps with it, she'll soon begin to recognize that what she's experiencing with Clyde isn't as simple and surface-level as she might believe.

Natasha is not an anomaly. She, like most of my clients, wanted to talk about the issue that brought her to therapy—whether to stay in her relationship or not. Peering too deeply into her past—her family dynamics, her programming and conditioning, her experiences from decades earlier—didn't seem relevant or useful or important. She knew an engagement was not far off (Clyde had been looking at engagement rings), so any time spent examining something other than this one particular relationship felt like a waste of time. To stay with Clyde or to go—that was the decision that was haunting her.

It made sense from her perspective, of course. Most people would rather stay focused on where they're headed, instead of where they've come from. But what Natasha didn't understand was that examining *only* Clyde was exactly what would keep her from clarity. Over the next couple of months in our work together, Natasha would not just examine her childhood and past relationships, she'd also examine quite a bit about both of her parents and her sister. Eventually a lot would begin to make sense—in regard to Clyde and to other issues she'd been grappling with for years.

. . .

It's worth the time to examine your family of origin . . . but this is not always easy. That's what we'll be doing together in the pages that follow. Because if we're not aware of the patterns we're working from, we are bound to repeat them in predictable—and often destructive—ways. Like Natasha did.

As with so many others, before her breakthrough, Natasha was committed to the story that her childhood was an ideal one. Her parents' marriage was still intact, and she'd grown up in a loving family system. "There's nothing to complain about. I had a pretty great childhood and I'd feel ridiculous trying to find a few things here and there to criticize, especially when so many others had it way harder than I did."

Natasha had fallen victim to both idealization and what I call *wound comparison*. She wouldn't give herself permission to acknowledge her story because "other people have had it worse." People in her own circle of acquaintance, in fact. She had a friend who experienced abuse from her father. She had another friend whose mother died when she was thirteen. And yet another friend whose brother stole all the family's money and gambled it away.

"Those are real issues. Those are real problems. That is real pain and trauma," she said. Her hurt and pain couldn't compare with the hurt and pain of friends and strangers alike. She didn't believe she had a right to feel.

Her use of the word *real* felt important to pay attention to. What I heard between the lines was: *My pain and my trauma are not as obvious. Can people still recognize that even if it's not as glaring? Can I recognize that for myself? Does my pain have room here?*

Because Natasha had pain in her past—I could hear it in her voice and see it in the corners of the stories she told me. But until she deemed that pain worthy of notice, we couldn't address it together.

Wound comparison is a distraction, regardless of whether you come in minimizing or maximizing. The focus moves you away from yourself—your story, your vulnerability, and ultimately your healing. It's also common, as Natasha did, to idealize your past. This is an attempt at protection. If you can continue seeing your family through a positive lens, you don't have to face the pain, feel like you're being disloyal to them, or appear unappreciative of the care and love that they *did* offer. And if the past isn't as secure as you make it out to be, there might be a lot of loss for what was or wasn't and fear for what your present and future might turn out to be.

This is a paradox that so many of us struggle with: thinking critically of our family of origin while also still honoring the love and effort that was there. It's difficult to hold two conflicting ideas in our heads at the same time. But if you can't look at your origin stories, if you can't look at your pain and trauma, if you get caught making what you experienced smaller or bigger than what it is, if you get stuck idealizing it, or if you get stuck intellectualizing it away, you run the very high risk of being a bystander in your own life.

Natasha would need to stop comparing and make space for her pain without any of the distractions. She'd need to acknowledge her true origin story. And she'd need to start by seeing the role she took on in keeping her family going.

Your Role in Your Family of Origin

Children are incredibly aware. They're constantly observing, watching, feeling, and sensing what's happening around them. They pay close attention to the emotional experiences of others, often offering a hug or a kiss to a parent or sibling they think is sad or upset. It's remarkable, really, to see children notice what so many adults often miss. Their intuition is still intact, and they're not plagued by constant distractions. They're present and attuned to their surroundings, and they haven't learned to cover up their pain or the pain of others with excuses or minimizing. They're not afraid to point out the pain they notice in others, either—and like most of us, they often instinctively want to solve any of the problems they sense.

That incredible sensitivity to pain and the impulse to make it go away often lead a child to step into playing a crucial role in the maintenance of a family, like offering family members emotional support or acting as a parental figure to a younger sibling. Maybe you were trying to distract your parents from the hard things that were happening in their lives, or maybe you just wanted to make things easier for your parents. For example, if you had a sibling with special needs, you may have noticed the stress and exhaustion in your parents and decided to take on the role of the low-maintenance child, the child who looks after themselves and does everything in their power not to add any more stress to a household hanging on by a thread. Attuned children see what is needed and then step into a role they believe will protect them or their family.

And here's the kicker: that role you took on way back when? It might still be conditioning your actions and responses today. It's one of the main ways your past continues to have a hold on you. You might unconsciously choose partners, friendships, or even jobs where you find yourself right back in a role you know all too well. If you were the family perfectionist, you might maintain your perfectionist tendencies in your adult relationships. If you were a caretaker to a parent or siblings, you might still feel compelled to look after everyone's needs. Maybe you were the lost child, the invisible one who made yourself small and quiet, and you struggle today to speak up. Or maybe you were the comic relief, and still see it as your role to amuse. But there's also a more subtle way that a childhood role comes along with you, which is when you find yourself rejecting the role you once were in as a child. If you were a confidant or an emotional support for a parent, you might notice that you want nothing to do with emotional care and intimacy with a partner. Any sign of emotional needs from a partner or friend might remind you of how draining being a support figure was for you growing up, so much so that you close yourself off to any and all connection, closeness, and vulnerability.

The role you took on may have been needed to keep a struggling family afloat. But it might not be needed today. In fact, that role you took on might be exactly what's *keeping* you from your healing. It might be keeping you from discovering, naming, and dealing with a deeper hurt, and thus from connection and closeness with a partner. That's what we learned as I dug deeper with Natasha about her hesitation to commit to her loving partner, Clyde.

As the weeks passed, Natasha continued to insist on her happy childhood. For several sessions I had been asking her about her fears around the proverbial "other shoe dropping" she anticipated in their relationship, her fear that one day Clyde would reveal something he had been hiding about himself. My questions about where the other shoe had dropped in her family and past relationships met no response, but when I asked Natasha whether she had ever hidden something herself, a door opened.

She shared that at age fifteen she had stumbled upon an email that had been left open on her father's computer. She was having some trouble with her own computer, and she needed to complete something for class the next day. She had asked her father if she could use his, to which he said yes.

"He must have not realized what he had left open," she said. Tears started to fill her eyes.

"The thread was right there. Right in front of me. I read every email between them. Every single one. I couldn't look away. It didn't make sense to me. Some woman, not my mother, was telling my father how much she loved him, how amazing the weekend had been, how she couldn't wait to spend their lives together. And my father was telling her the same things back. This had been going on for years. Years. And no one knew. My dad walked in on me. I just stared at him with tears in my eyes and started to bawl. My mother was gone on a work trip that week and my sister was at basketball practice. He looked at me and said, 'Please don't tell your mother. I promise I'll cut it off.' We never talked about it again, and I never told my mother. He stopped the affair—I would check his email and phone regularly to make sure of it. He let me do this. I think it was our unspoken way of making sure our 'agreement' stayed intact."

She paused and shook her head. She had been looking down while she shared this with me. Her gaze rose, and she found my eyes.

"What a heavy burden to carry," I said steadily to her. "What a secret to hold for over two decades. I can only imagine the pain, the confusion, and the questioning you've done."

Natasha had held the secret. She had played her role magnificently. She'd kept the secret so well, including from herself, that it would almost be forgotten, oddly absorbed in such a way in order to allow for her family to continue to function in the way they always did: happy, connected, loving—as if nothing was wrong.

No wonder she believed her childhood was great. Natasha's role as secret-keeper had covered up and distracted them all from any underlying pain and sadness. But it was the very success of Natasha's role-playing that allowed the past to tighten its grip on her and prevent her from finding a more constructive way forward.

Trading Authenticity for Attachment

When you were a child, there were probably endless moments when you were either asked or encouraged to be a little more of this and a little less of that to get love, connection, validation, safety, or affirmation from your parents and caretakers. You may have received messaging from your parents, messaging they thought was harmless, that was actually asking you to become less of who you were. And guess what you did when you were a kid? You probably went along with it. You want to know why? Because you are wired for attachment. Because attachment is necessary for your survival. And because your need to be loved, wanted, chosen, protected, prioritized, and safe trumps everything else.

But just as necessary as your need for attachment is your need for authenticity. To be authentic is to be free to be and to feel; it's to be fully revealed to yourself and to those you let into your intimate space. Authenticity is at the core of our existence. Without it, an internal death takes place.

Authenticity and attachment are both powerful needs. Yet, as Dr. Gabor Maté, a trauma and addiction specialist, says, "When authenticity threatens attachment, attachment trumps authenticity." What a thought to consider that so many of us must trade one lifeline for another: *To stay connected to you, I must leave and abandon me, or to stay true to myself, I must choose to disconnect from you.* And what a thought to think about tiny humans, including you, who needed to make that decision time and time again.

As children, we *do* trade our authenticity for attachment. Of course we do; it's the more important lifeline. Perfect grades make Dad happy. Being quieter makes Mom less irritable. Losing weight gets you attention. Being fine means your parents are less stressed out. Acting out means Dad stops hurting your sister. Agreeing keeps the peace. Helping Mom makes her less sad. You learned to adjust yourself to make sure your parents didn't abandon, reject, hate, criticize, judge, or disown you. And as adults, we sadly engage in this, too. But it's because we're conditioned to do it. It's because we've learned that our worthiness, belonging, prioritization, trust, and safety are given when we shift and change ourselves to accommodate others.

It is here, in your origin story with attachment and authenticity, where you first learn to engage in a recurring self-betrayal. It is here where you learn to abandon your true self for attachment. It is here where you begin to shapeshift, transforming who you are in order to get what you believe you need.

Take that in for a moment. You've been convinced that being someone other than who you are is the only way you get the things you crave the most. *If I become who you need me to be, I can guarantee myself love, connection, approval, safety, and validation.* It's a form of self-protection, and you tried your darndest to accommodate. But becoming a successful shapeshifter isn't actually a victory. It doesn't actually reap the benefit that you want. Even if you get validation for getting the As, scoring the hat trick, or being less emotional, deep down you know what's up. You see through it and know that when validation is given because of inauthenticity, it can't be trusted. No wonder we turn into adults who are insecure, unsure, and doubting of ourselves and others. No wonder it's so hard to show up authentically and trust that another will love, choose, respect, and honor you.

Natasha's story provides an excellent example. She'd become an extraordinary shapeshifter. She'd avoided the pain of her father's infidelity so that her family could go on. Yet victories don't get much hollower. She'd carried that heavy weight for so long that she no longer knew how to honor her own pain, her own sadness, her own loss. She'd traded her authentic self for attachment to her father, who needed his secret kept, and to her mother, who was kept in the dark. That trade was robbing her of freedom, of resiliency, of being able to dance in the ebb and flow that relationships inevitably present and relationally walk with her partner toward healing. Natasha was sitting on the sidelines of her own life, letting the unresolved issues of her past dictate her life story and intrude upon her relationships and healing.

Our Past Is the Key to Our Present—and Our Future

I know it can be tempting to keep your eyes on the prize. I know you might want to stay facing forward, but I'm going to need you to be more of a swivel head. The things from the past, all that family stuff, it matters . . . a lot. If you want to heal your relationships with yourself and others, then understanding your origin stories is necessary. Your unhealed and unresolved past is directing your life today, but it doesn't have to continue to do so.

Legacies, family secrets, and fears and insecurities get passed down the generational chain. Some of those things are overtly offered and chosen—like cherished holiday rituals, family mantras, or Tuesday taco night. But other traditions that get handed down are unhealthy, even insidious. A woman who becomes increasingly critical of her daughter's weight in the same way her mother criticized her. A father whose patience begins to shorten when his children don't meet his unrealistic expectations, even though he hated his father for the rigidity and rules by which he felt controlled. An affair that is not to be spoken of for fear of judgment by others in the community, or the death of a young child that is never fully acknowledged and grieved.

When Natasha found her father's emails, the experience left her with both a doubt of others and, just as damaging, a doubt of herself. Although she wasn't consciously aware of this, Natasha began to live life with distrust. She didn't know what she could and couldn't believe. She was drawn to "good" people, safe people, people she would describe as honest, kind, thoughtful, and considerate, but no matter how consistent they were, she was always expecting for something to go wrong. Her way of coping was to end relationships prematurely; then she wouldn't have to wait for the other shoe to drop in the same way she did decades earlier with her father.

This wasn't obvious to Natasha. She had never told another soul the story of discovering her father's betrayal. It was locked inside her until she spoke it out loud to me. Over the next many weeks, Natasha would understand that her doubts about Clyde, her concern that something was "just off," were extensions of this massive rupture she experienced with her father. The avoidance and secrecy that was subtly asked of her by her father kept her stuck, and the continued avoidance and secrecy that she maintained with herself kept her choosing exceptional partners whom she believed would ultimately somehow deceive her. It was only when we delved deep into her origin healing practice that she was able to release herself from her past and find a happier ending and a healthier path.

For many, and maybe you, we first have to come to terms with the fact that this work of exploring your origins—though vital—isn't always easy. The idea of looking back at your childhood can be downright daunting. It might scare you to think about what you might find, it can feel overwhelming to consider whether you'll be able to handle what you do uncover, and it can feel like a distraction away from the very important issues at hand.

The reality is, most of us are more inclined to wait until we're in crisis. And what I can tell you from my professional experience is that couples and individuals generally wait longer than they ought to before seeking support.

Whether you're in a relationship or not, you might notice yourself bargaining with yourself and looking for a simpler, easier way out.

I should be able to figure this out on my own.

29

If I go to therapy, more bad things are going to get uncovered.

My family did the best they could, and I don't want to hate them by digging up unnecessary things.

But what if the digging into your origin story could yield the relief and the exact answers you've been looking for all along?

2

NAMING YOUR WOUND

Every single day people like Natasha go to therapy for the first time wanting to talk about the problems they're facing right now. I've had hundreds of first sessions with individuals, couples, and families, and that first session almost always sounds something like: *We just keep fighting about the same things and never have any resolution. Or, we're not connected sexually. Or, I'm so stressed about trying to find out my future and what I should be doing. Or, I just need to stop trying to get my mom to see my perspective.*

Most people want a solution as quickly as possible. They want to get from point A (distress) to point B (relief) as fast as they can. *How do we stop fighting like this? Can you help us find a solution?* Or better yet, *Can't you just tell us who's right and who's wrong?* And here's the thing: We can create some rules and strategy around how to fight, how to speak to one another more kindly in heated moments, how to express gratitude, and how to get each to see the other's perspective on the dirty dishes, the in-laws, or the overspending. And maybe in that therapy session you *do* feel a sense of relief, as if you've made some real progress.

But let me tell you what almost always happens next. That same couple comes back the following week sharing a story that sounds pretty much like the previous one. The young woman who wants to stop trying to get her mom to understand her had another conversation with her mom that went south, yet again. And that couple trying out new ways to connect sexually keeps feeling more hopeless when their attempts fall flat.

I'm going to give you a shortcut early on in this book, okay? It's simple but important. You might already have a sense about what it is based on what you've already read, but in case there's any confusion, this is a good place for me to clear any possible misunderstanding.

Here it goes: *There is likely much more going on under the surface than the issue you first come into a therapist's office to discuss.*

If you're going to make long-lasting, integrated change, you must understand what's under the hood. And under that hood are origin stories and unresolved pain from your family that need attention if what's happening present day is going to have a chance at repair and relief. If you can't move with ease past what's playing out presently, there's a reason for that. Origin healing work requires us to investigate our families of origin, to discover or identify those pain points, and to name what was previously left unnamed.

The Origins of *You*

So where do we begin? We begin where *you* begin. Maybe not *that* far back, but we're going to rewind pretty far. You're about to learn about the origins of you.

We begin with your family of origin. This is the family system in which you grew up, and in this system are the people whom you were and maybe still are emotionally connected to. As a note, I'll use *family of origin* and *family system* interchangeably throughout these pages. The people in your family of origin laid the foundation for your beliefs, values, and identity, whether they were related to you by blood or not. It's where you get your first education on just about everything from love to conflict to criticism. Your family of origin taught you about yourself, about how to engage with others, and what to expect out of relationships. You might have one family system, or if you're like me (with divorced parents and separate family dynamics in each), you have two. You might have even more than that.

For many, your parents and siblings were your primary guides. But for many others, a family of origin includes grandparents, stepparents and stepsiblings, adoptive family, foster families, or an aunt or uncle who moved in with you. I've had clients who grew up with nannies they spent more time with than their own kin, and clients who would go to their neighbor's home after school until ten P.M., when their parent returned from work. *These* people are easily considered a part of your family of origin.

And if you grew up with multiple family systems, you'll want to look at each. Learning to be part of and navigate multiple families is no easy task. They each offered you their own specific education. You may have received opposing messages around work ethic, the importance of education, or proper behavior for children from each dynamic. You may have had to abide by different rules between homes—like how much television you were allowed to watch, when you had to go to bed, what types of foods you could eat, or what kinds of chores you were expected to do. And you may have learned to exist differently between the homes if differing socioeconomic statuses or religious beliefs were involved.

But what also might have been different is where you experienced pain or sadness or ease and joy. You might have felt worthy in one family and not in another. You may have felt safe in one home but scared in another. And you may have felt prioritized with one parent but not with another. Navigating multiple families of origin is rarely an easy task. But understanding your different experiences is one worth noting *before* we dive in, so you remember to look in multiple places for these origin stories, not just in your primary home base.

An origin story is the story about your firsts. The first time you were taught something, the first time you observed and witnessed something, the first time you were told something that had an impact on you, and crucially for our purposes, the first time you experienced harm. And although your firsts, no matter what they are, are important, what really leaves an imprint is the first time something profoundly painful happens, something life-changing happens, or when someone or something asks you to change who you are—even if the actual memory of what happened has long been buried.

I want to note that although the first education you get about love, communication, boundaries, and other things comes from your family of origin, origin stories are not always birthed in your family. They don't even necessarily originate in your childhood! You will find origin stories and influences from society, media, religion, teachers, coaches, and past romantic relationships. These stories can be written in your teen years, young adult life, or even just a short time ago— whenever you encounter something for the first time. Origin stories are often (but not always) childhood stories. We're continually writing and rewriting the narrative of our lives.

Now you might think you know a lot of this already—rightfully so, given the fact that you're the only one who has lived *your* life. But every single time I rewind and journey back, I learn something new about myself. I see myself through a new lens, and I think you might, too. So let's dive into an initial set of questions that help you begin the process.

Your Origin Questions: Getting Started

When I begin my work with clients, it's necessary that I learn about what it was like for them growing up. I want to know about their families of origin, the relational dynamics (past and present), the qualities of each family member, the experiences and observations the client had growing up, and so much more. In this exploration we also begin to identify what they wanted or needed as kids and didn't get. Tough stuff, I know, but so crucial in understanding present-day sensitivities.

As you explore, you might remember traits or characteristics of your family members that you haven't thought about in a long time. You might reflect on how things changed in your family after a particular event, or how behaviors and beliefs have been passed down generationally. Familiarizing yourself with this part of the system is important. It helps give you a more comprehensive look at your family of origin, your relationships with them, and their relationships with one another. It helps you begin to identify patterns.

I'd encourage you to keep a journal close by as you read through this book and work through the exercises. You might jot something down that deeply resonates with you, and you might want to journal your responses to the many questions you'll be asked along the way. Take good care of yourself as you begin to explore.

Although some of the questions I ask might differ client to client, I'll almost always ask the following:

- Who did you have around you growing up?
- How did the adults treat each other?
- In what ways did they express love to one another?
- Describe your father to me—both who he was as an individual and who he was as a father to you. Share the things you admired, the things you judged, what you liked and disliked.
- Describe your mother to me—both who she was as an individual and who she was as a mother to you. Share the things you admired, the things you judged, what you liked and disliked.

35

- If you had any stepparents or other parental figures in your life, please answer the same questions.
- Were there any events that happened that changed the way the adults treated one another or treated you? If so, share with me what those events were and what shifted.
- Were there any mental health challenges that anyone in your family faced?
- How were those addressed or not addressed?
- Did infidelity, betrayal, major transitions, loss, or death take place in the family?
- How did that impact the family?
- What is something you wish your father understood about you? What is something you wish your mother understood about you?
- If they understood those things, what do you believe would have been different about your relationship with them?
- What did you crave as a child?
- Describe your relationship with each of your siblings, if any.
- If you could tell your father one thing and there would be absolutely no consequence at all, what would that be?
- If you could tell your mother one thing and there would be absolutely no consequences at all, what would that be?
- What is your favorite memory from childhood?
- What is your most painful memory from childhood?

Answering these questions takes time, curiosity, openness, courage, and vulnerability, but when you do this work, you offer yourself valuable insight and context for both your past and your present experiences.

Revealing the Wound

As you dive into your memories of the past, you're likely going to come face-to-face with things that feel particularly challenging and emotional. This is completely normal. Origin healing work requires us to identify and name our *origin wound*, the unhealed and festering pain from the past that you have yet to fully acknowledge in your life. Revealing and naming this wound is one of the biggest steps you'll take toward your healing.

When I hear the word *wound*, I always think first about a physical wound. Remember scraping your knee or elbow as a kid? A parent might clean it up for you, put a Band-Aid over it, and remind you to let some air get in there to help it heal. Eventually a scab would form over it. But then you'd bump it on the side of a table or you'd pick at the scab (as kids do), only to have it start bleeding again. That wound would become raw once more and you'd experience the physical pain as if it were the first time.

Emotional wounds are similar. They form because you have a painful experience that affects you on an emotional and psychological level. There might not be anything to show for it, like a scab, but it has lasting effects, effects that run deep. Those emotional wounds, like physical ones, get poked and prodded and become raw again throughout life.

Yet unlike physical wounds, where the body naturally heals itself, emotional ailments that are left unattended don't mend on their own. I'm sorry to say, time alone does *not* heal all wounds. It might make some lighter and easier, but deep emotional pain needs your attention, your presence, your emotion, and your intentional energy. And even then, they still need your care. Wounds don't disappear; they just fade.

That's why you can't just look the other way. Looking for your origin wounds isn't meant to send you on a wild-goose chase; it's meant to direct you to the source of your pain. And because for so many, emotional wounding has its origins in the family system, we begin by looking there.

What You Wanted Most Was . . .

I'd like to start our work together with one of the most important questions a therapist has ever asked me, a question that has always stayed with me: What did you want most as a child and not get?

Hang on. Don't blow past this; actually take a moment to answer the question. I know it may elicit a lot of emotion. And I know it requires a lot of bravery and vulnerability to sit with that question and answer it honestly. But there's some important information in your response.

What you most wanted in your family system but didn't get was likely something you really could have used. Maybe you wanted to feel worthy even when you weren't bringing home perfect grades. Maybe you wanted to belong, to feel accepted and loved for your differences. Maybe you wanted to feel prioritized. Maybe you wanted to trust that the adults were being honest with you and not hiding things from you, or to feel protected in a home that often felt scary.

When those things don't happen, a wound is born.

In other words, you might have a worthiness wound. Or a belonging wound. Or a prioritization wound—or a trust wound or a safety wound. We'll discuss all these in much more detail in part 2. But for now, just know that when you didn't get what you wanted most, the things you really could have used, there is pain there that needs to be examined.

This isn't an invitation to look for the bad. Your parents may have cared deeply, but they may have lacked the tools to meet your emotional needs. Also, please note that you don't have to have the worst story in the world to have a wound. This is about your honoring your own experience without tampering with it, without distorting it or explaining it away. This work is about naming the loss and witnessing the parts of the self that need your attention. When we do this successfully, we begin to reveal our wounds to ourselves.

Remember how in order to keep the peace in her family, Natasha kept her father's secret but also was unable to name her own pain? How she pushed down her discovery of the adulterous emails to save her parents' relationship? Yet whether she admitted it or not, Natasha's vision of her father—a story about him and her parents' marriage—had been shattered in that moment of discovery. She had been convinced her parents were happy together, that they were in love. She had been convinced that her father was a good, honorable man. He was home by six every night, and he loved spending time with his wife and kids. He would do loving things for his wife, and he genuinely seemed to enjoy his family.

Natasha couldn't reconcile what she had witnessed, what she had experienced, what she believed to be true about him with the same man who had been having an affair for years. Her life, her joyful memories—they were all being questioned. She had been duped, really betrayed, in the same way that she believed her mother and sister had been. In that instant, her relationship with her father fundamentally changed, as did her relationship with her mother and sister.

Her trust wound was born.

In the next many months after Natasha's discovery of her wound and of what she most wanted, we co-explored her childhood, this rupture, and its lasting effects. When she named her trust wound for what it was, when she acknowledged that what she'd most wanted as a child was trust and that instead she'd been betrayed, it revealed to her a whole new part of herself that she now knew needed attention and for the first time opened up the genuine possibility of healing.

. . .

What I wanted most as a child was to know that there was room for me not to be okay. I wished that I knew and trusted that I didn't have to fake it and pretend, that there was room for my struggle and pain, too, and that I didn't need to be a well-adjusted kid who was taking things in stride. I wish that that permission had been offered to me by my parents. I wanted to be truly seen and understood by them, not seen and understood for the version I was presenting. I needed them to see through the facade. I wanted *them* to be responsible for their emotions and their emotional regulation so that I didn't feel pressure to be responsible for these on their behalf. I didn't want to always think about having to say the right thing so as not to upset them or hurt their feelings. *This* is what I had wished was different.

Okay, now your turn.

You might know exactly what you wanted as a child—or in an important adult relationship—that you didn't get. It might be so obvious to you that you don't think much about it at all. But if the answer isn't as clear, you might need to slow down and really consider what it is you needed but didn't get. Or maybe we change the question up a bit to this: If something could have been different about your childhood, what would it be?

If you have something, beautiful. If you've got nothing, that's okay, too. Trust the timing of what will be revealed.

How We Conceal Our Wounds

A favorite question of therapists around the world is what we call the *constraint question*. Instead of asking why you do or don't do something, we ask you what *keeps* you from doing or not doing something. What's the constraint?

When it comes to naming or revealing your wounds to yourself, the same question applies: What keeps you from seeing your wound? It turns out, most of us use one or many creative methods to block ourselves from seeing, revealing, or spending time with the wound. Sometimes we do this consciously and sometimes not.

HIDING

One of the ways we cover up our wounds is by hiding, something I was skilled at. You may have been able to guess that, since I did it so well as a child, literally hiding in a closet with my mother. But that skill set just got stronger and stronger through my teen years and early twenties. I hid *everything* vulnerable. Boyfriends would do things I didn't like, and I'd pretend it was fine. Friends would take advantage of me, and I'd blow it off as nothing. In every situation, I'd say I was good when in fact I wasn't.

I was so good at hiding that you would never have known how scared and insecure I was.

Hiding does a good job of convincing the outside world of something very different from what's happening in your inside world. But by hiding your hurt, pain, fears, and insecurity from others, you exist in the world inauthentically. Like my client Aazam, who struggles with depression as the result of a safety wound. Just getting through the day is a trial sometimes, but instead of telling any of her friends about it when she hits a rough patch, she just stays in on weekends and self-isolates. Why? So that her friends don't think she's boring or a downer and drop her. Or Dom, who struggles with a worthiness wound and is so ashamed of the house he grew up in that he has never taken a partner to his parents' home for fear of what they might think. Hiding might make you feel safe in the short term, but the result is that you're not fully showing up in the relationships that matter most to you.

AVOIDING

Another way we cover up is to avoid. You avoid your wound by making sure you don't ever come close to it. You put as much space between you and your wound as you can. Maybe you fear rejection or intimacy, so instead of facing the wound, you choose to *never* date. Or maybe you're afraid of failure, so you've never applied for a promotion. After all, you don't ever have to reveal your wound to yourself if it never gets touched or even looked at. That's what avoidance protects against.

PERFORMING

Some of us cover up wounds by constantly performing. Performers can put on a great show. You can be a perfectionist and make it seem like your life is perfectly put together. This keeps you protected from having to face your fears, doubts, and insecurities. If you successfully perform, you don't have to face the pain. This was true for Jennie, who worked a ninety-hour workweek just to impress her boss and colleagues. It worked—her performance was exceptional—but somehow the kudos in her professional life weren't feeling as fulfilling as they once had. For years, she'd used her performance in her professional life as a barometer of her success. After all, if she could always be celebrated at work, she never had to feel less than and not good enough, feelings she lived with in childhood.

PLEASING

We also cover up our wounds by becoming the person who pleases others above all else. When you successfully please, you're working hard at never letting someone down, and you work tirelessly at keeping it up. Roz, a typical people pleaser, tells me that they show up for every single event for all their friends. They never turn down an invite, and they're always the first one to show up and the last one to leave. They focus on maintaining approval, as being liked keeps Roz from having to face feeling like they weren't liked or wanted growing up.

Letting yourself be vulnerable is a scary and challenging commitment. But it's one we make to free ourselves from staying stuck. You can't heal if you're hiding your wounds from yourself; you can't heal if you're avoiding acknowledging your pain.

And you can't heal if you continue to perform for or please others as a way to distract yourself from your wound. Just take that in for a moment.

You can't make changes in your life if you cover up your own hurt and pain from yourself. You can't live differently if you block yourself from the things that need your attention. Doing this will keep you stuck. And I get it, you might not be ready to go *there* (sharing and revealing your pain to others or even fully feeling yourself). But see if you can make a little bit of room for yourself to feel as you read this book. It's just you and me here. No need to share this with anyone else if you don't want to.

The Cost of Covering Our Wounds

We cover up our wounds because they're hard to face. They're emotional and raw, and they put a spotlight on things from the past that were hurtful and harmful. It's easier to just get on with life than to go *there*. If we could move on without acknowledging the wound, people would probably sign up for that.

But simply moving on doesn't work. You want to know why?

Because wounds don't just go away. They don't take up less space because you turn away from them. They don't mend on their own because you ignore them. They don't heal because you avoid them.

They are persistent because they want to be healed.

If you try to cover up a wound, it will find a way to grab your attention. In fact, it's been *trying* to grab your attention in ways that you might not even register—ways that are probably more common than you think. In fact, a wound may have tried to grab your attention this last week or this last month, but you just might not know what to look out for.

Perhaps you've found yourself *becoming* your parent unconsciously, like when you criticize your partner in the same way you saw your mom criticize your dad, or when you blow up at your partner just as your parents blew up at each other. Or in other cases, you might be so scared about repeating your parents' patterns that you do everything in your power *not* to be like them. This is a healthy impulse in some situations, but one that still has you making decisions driven by fear—like avoiding conflict at all costs, a decision that might keep things peaceful on the surface but prevents you from ever voicing your frustrations or concerns.

Does any of this sound familiar? You've likely already seen these behaviors play out in your friendships, your work relationships, or your current or past partnerships (don't worry, you're not the only one raising your hand here). These behaviors, whether they are conscious or unconscious, are all great indicators that an origin wound is trying to get your attention.

REACTIVITY

Reactivity is one of the greatest indicators that you have a wound. When you have a strong reaction to something, that reaction is sounding an alarm. Your inner self knows *something* about what's happening, and your reactivity is letting you know that you don't like what's going on, that you feel uncomfortable or threatened, or that you're in danger.

Sometimes reactivity is because deep down you feel something very familiar is showing up. A partner looks down at his phone while you're sharing something vulnerable with him and you storm off. His distraction reminds you of your parent, who didn't prioritize you while you were growing up. A friend cancels plans on you for the third time and you tell her off. Her lack of consideration for you reminds you of your parent, who promised things but never followed through.

We've all been there. When I asked my Instagram community what makes them reactive, there were hundreds of entries. Some of their answers were: being criticized, being dismissed, being blamed, avoiding accountability, being told I'm too sensitive, being interrupted, not feeling heard, being rejected, and more. Why do we overreact? We'll be exploring this further as we explore our different wounds, but for now, the key point is that strong reactions are like a flag in the sand, indicating that if you dig a bit, you'll find an origin wound that still needs tending.

BLOWING THINGS OUT OF PROPORTION

Another sign of a wound just below the surface is when you blow things out of proportion, or when there's a seeming inconsistency between a blowup and whatever provoked it. Mahika enthusiastically offered to cook for a woman she'd been dating for a couple of months. But when the woman showed up at her door empty-handed and plopped down on her sofa as Mahika continued cooking, her feelings shifted. Her guest was engaging, talking about the events of her day and asking Mahika questions. But Mahika could feel herself start to spiral internally: *I can't believe you're so inconsiderate. Why aren't you asking if you can help? You're just taking advantage of me. I'm sick of taking care of others.* And soon enough, the internal becomes external. "Why'd you even come over if you're not interested in spending time with me?" The tears began to flow. This, for many, would be a confusing exchange. The invited person likely had no clue what had just happened. She was present and happy to be there. But Mahika was having a big reaction to something that both was and wasn't happening in this moment.

When someone or you has a reaction that appears to be bigger than what you believe is appropriate, consider that in this reaction lies a rich and complex history—one that would help make this current moment make sense, or at the very minimum give it context. In this case, Mahika had grown up with an alcoholic parent who would plop down on the sofa, make demands, and always expect to be taken care of. When her date showed up empty-handed and didn't offer to help, Mahika unconsciously flashed back to those angry feelings of being taken advantage of. Deep down, she was experiencing her negative feelings from the past, not the present, and having a strong reaction because of an unhealed prioritization wound, which we'll discuss in more detail in chapter 5.

DYSFUNCTIONAL PATTERNS

Another way a covered or unnamed wound shows through is in repeat behaviors and choices that don't support your emotional, physical, mental, relational, or spiritual well-being. You might keep choosing the same types of partners time and time again: partners who always cheat on you or hide something from you, or ones who are emotionally disengaged or unwilling to commit. Or you might have promised yourself that you wouldn't keep having one-night stands because every single time you do, you feel awful the next day . . . but you find yourself out engaging in that same behavior no matter how many times you promise yourself you won't. Or maybe you keep draining your bank account to "keep up" financially with your friends, just to find yourself stressed out about how to pay the rent at the end of the month.

Do any of these sound like you?

These are all dysfunctional patterns. The behavior ranges from procrastinating, playing mind games when dating, lying, excusing hurtful or harmful behavior, getting roped into useless arguments, engaging in negative self-talk, to giving more than you receive (non-reciprocal relationships). What they all have in common is that they reflect an unacknowledged wound.

SABOTAGE

One of the most dysfunctional patterns involves sabotaging ourselves and our relationships. When you engage in sabotage, you test others, usually unconsciously, with the hope of either continuing to hide and thus reinforcing your wound or bringing everything that needs healing to the surface.

One of the most common ways I see people test or sabotage a relationship is through infidelity. Now there are certainly many reasons why people cheat, but I've worked with countless individuals who have engaged in cheating as a form of sabotage. *If I cheat, you'll find out, and then you'll leave me because I'm undeserving of this relationship anyway.* This reinforces a wound that says you're unworthy of love, intimacy, or partnership—ultimately suggesting that you're unworthy of being chosen.

But sabotage can also be an attempt at correcting the wound. The correction might go something like this: *If I cheat, you'll find out. It will blow up our relationship, but maybe we can start to talk about why*

I feel so undeserving of you as my partner. Maybe we can talk about why I don't feel like I'm good enough for you. And maybe from there you'll help me see and understand why I actually am a valuable and important person in your life, deserving of a future with you. Whew, I know. And yet this is more common than you might think.

GIVING ADVICE YOU CAN'T TAKE

Finally, there's a maybe less expected sign of a wound fighting to surface: that of the person who gives advice but can't take it. Here I know a lot of hands are going to go up. I'm fairly certain that most of us have done this at some point in our lives. You tell a friend how he should stop talking to his ex, but when yours reaches out, you text back immediately. You offer your sibling advice on how to mentally prep for a job interview, but you struggle to feel confident yourself when you're in the same position. You promote self-love for others on your Instagram page, but you struggle to find anything you like about yourself behind closed doors.

If you give advice that you struggle to take or act on yourself, this is letting you know that there's something unresolved playing out. Maybe you can't take the self-love advice and offerings you give to others because you grew up believing no one loved you. What we preach but can't practice is just another indicator that we must slow down and get curious about what is unhealed.

All of the above are not the only ways a wound emerges to grab your attention, but they are the most consistent signs I've seen that let me and my clients know there is more to examine there. If you see any of these signs in yourself, I can almost guarantee you, there is more to uncover.

Naming the Wound

You'll notice that in this book I tell a lot of stories. I do this because many of us are so skilled at covering up the wounds that sometimes the simplest way to access our own is to see it through someone else's story. The stories of others can serve as illustrations and often provoke moments of recognition. Reading these stories and doing the exercises will help you bring to the surface what you've either buried or are struggling to recognize. Not every one of the varied stories I recount or wounds I identify will be yours to name. But here and throughout part 2, I hope the stories of others and their discoveries will help elicit your own aha moments and support you in your own naming process. Let's start with my client Monica.

I started working with Monica when she was forty-one and had come to me with sadness about fertility complications. She had done everything in her power to set herself up for success, but nothing was working. This was debilitating and emotionally exhausting; getting pregnant was all she thought about.

She praised her new husband, Michael, whom she described as supportive, loving, and invested, very different from her first husband, who was checked out and a "functioning addict." But the night prior, Michael and she had had a blowout fight in which things started out bad and escalated from there. As she recounted the argument to me, Monica was clearly ashamed of her behavior.

"I knew that Michael was going to a dinner after work. He told me about this over a week ago and it was on the calendar. But when he got home around eleven, I picked a fight over nothing and even took his phone and threw it across the room. I'm so embarrassed."

This reaction was a big one, and it didn't make sense—even to her. "I don't know why I did that. He didn't do anything wrong. He came home after the dinner and communicated with me throughout the night. What's wrong with me?" she asked.

Monica's disproportionate reaction was a five-alarm fire of a wound that was trying to grab her attention. We decided to explore further to see if we could identify whether a wound might have been activated for her the night before.

Monica's parents had gotten pregnant with her when they were in their early twenties. "Dad was never around, and Mom had no idea how to be a mom. No one took care of me. No one guided me or supported me with anything. No one seemed to remember that I even existed. I had to figure everything out on my own: from doing my homework to feeding myself to getting to and from school. It was awful."

This was the moment to ask that important question my therapist once asked me. "What did you want most as a child and not get?" I asked her.

"Everything," she said.

In many ways it was true, but it was also a deflection. I sat silent, allowing her a moment to tune into herself a bit more.

Tears started to well up in her eyes. "I just wanted to know that I mattered enough for someone to pay attention, for someone to be curious and ask how I was. It was exhausting figuring everything out on my own. Is that so much to ask?"

It wasn't, of course, but that didn't change her experience.

"What happened yesterday during the day?" I asked.

"I had work and a doctor's appointment."

"How did the doctor's appointment go? Was this your fertility doctor?"

"Yes. It wasn't great. I got some pretty shocking and upsetting news. The doctor doesn't think I'll be able to carry to term and is suggesting that we consider surrogacy."

This was a lot for her to process.

In earlier sessions I had learned that Nick, her first husband, prioritized his alcoholism. He would forget important details, would miss events that had been scheduled on the calendar for months, and could rarely offer a helping hand because he was either hung over or drinking. That marriage so obviously repeated the dynamic from her childhood that it was bound to fail, and fail it did.

But Monica had been deliberate in choosing Michael. "No red flags," she said. "He loves me and makes plans for us. We have so much fun together and love adventure." She was certain there was no pattern playing out here.

"How does Michael feel about surrogacy?" I asked.

"I don't know. I didn't tell him."

"Oh? Is there a reason you haven't?"

"We just don't talk about the fertility issues all that much. He wants a baby so badly, and it's hard on him. In his first marriage, it was a deal breaker. His ex decided she didn't want to have children, and it ended the marriage. So I guess I try to shield him from what's happening. He knows I'll go to my appointments and do what I need to do, you know? I'm responsible like that."

"I do know," I said. "I know that you've always taken care of things on your own. And I'm wondering if sitting with this news last night, by yourself, activated something? Even though you knew that Michael had a dinner, I'm wondering if what you were really craving was for him to ask you how you were doing. And for you to not have to figure the next steps out all on your own."

We sat in silence for what felt like minutes. Her whole body shifted. She dropped her face into her hands and started to sob. Of course Michael had had no idea what had happened at the doctor's appointment. He didn't even know she'd *had* a doctor's appointment. In this context, the puzzle pieces of Monica's shocking response all started to come together.

Michael and Monica had a beautiful marriage in many ways, but

Monica couldn't be the only one leading the charge. They both wanted a child, and that required both of them to participate. She needed to feel his effort, his interest, his commitment. Her big, confusing reaction led us straight to a childhood wound (a prioritization wound that we'll discuss in more detail in chapter 5) that was being activated by Michael's lack of support, guidance, and contribution.

It's all too common to become self-critical, even disgusted with yourself, when you've hit the "here we go again" button one too many times. Like Monica, you might ask yourself, *What's wrong with me? Why do I keep doing this? Why can't I change this pattern? Why do I keep choosing these types of people? Why do I always lose it with my mom? Why am I not over this yet?* But these questions just spin you in circles without any clear direction. In fact, you do things for a very good reason. Your inner self is trying to protect you; it just needs your awareness to help move you out of your old patterns onto a new healthier, more constructive path. First you must uncover and name the wound that prompts your recurring patterns.

You've picked up this book because your and others' behavior had you on a path that needed some attention. Here you'll learn that to get on a healthier road you'll need to examine your origin stories and the wounds that originated when what you wanted most in your family wasn't available to you. You'll learn to ask questions like "What's familiar about this?" "When was the first time I experienced this?" "With whom did I experience it?" and "What from my past is showing up in this moment?" You will get into the practice of noticing your dysfunctional behaviors, and then looking to both connect to and understand the origin wounds that are showing up and needing your attention.

You'll learn how to name your wound and how to witness and honor your pain from the past, grieve alongside of that pain, and then pivot, finding ways to create change in your life and your patterns. This is the Origin Healing Practice you'll learn more about in the next chapter.

As we close out this chapter, I want to remind you of something important: Your life isn't out to get you. It's out to be healed. Your wounds don't want to harm you; they're tugging at you because you deserve relief. The journey of reclaiming yourself and taking charge of your own life is a long one, an ongoing process. But in recognizing the effects of your origin wounds and working to lessen the impact they have on your behaviors today, you can begin traveling down the necessary path of healing.

So the question is, on a scale from "Let's do this!" to Brené Brown at her first therapy session, how ready are you?

PART II

OUR WOUNDS AND THEIR ORIGINS

3

I WANT TO FEEL WORTHY

At an event many years ago, I offered the attendees the prompt "I'm unworthy because . . ." The room was quiet and still. They slowly and bravely started to call out their own truths. A voice from the back quietly spoke.

"I'm not slim enough."

Another voice offered, "I repeat the same mistakes."

And another: "I'm not successful."

And another: "I don't have a career and rely on my husband's money."

They kept coming:

"Because there are more attractive people out there."

"I'm lazy."

"I'm obsessed with my work."

"I'm too emotional."

"My family is too much."

"I can't do anything right."

"I'm not smart enough."

"I never open up."

"I'm too sensitive."

"I'm fat."

"I'm divorced."

"I've hurt people."

"I'm still single."

"People leave me."

Tears started to fill the eyes of the attendees. As they heard the other participants' reasons, heads were shaking no. This exercise offered a sense of togetherness and solidarity—*we've all got something, and we're in this together.* We could have probably done many rounds of this, but it was understood that this was enough.

When you don't feel worthy at your core, you don't feel deserving of good things. You don't feel like you are good enough—*as you are*—to receive love, attention, presence, and commitment. You might struggle to believe that you are allowed to have joy, ease, and partnership. A worthiness wound might mean that you have a hard time believing and trusting that you are valuable and valued, that you are deserving of the things you crave in the world without needing to perform or be perfect to receive them.

Deep down, many people struggle with this. You believe you're too dysfunctional or too lazy or just plain undeserving of a relationship. You ask yourself questions like: *How could anyone love me if my own parents didn't? Am I still worthy of love if I'm not successful? Will anyone want to be with me? Do I deserve to have anyone choose me if I'm not a good person?* The list goes on.

I'm unworthy because . . . The answers seem endless.

But what if the entire premise is false? What if you *are* worthy and deserving of good things? What if you do deserve love and joy and strong partnerships?

After all, you are not born unworthy, so what is it that happens between birth and this moment that makes you question it?

Like the seminar attendees, you may be ready to label yourself as unworthy. In fact, hearing that you are indeed worthy, simply by having been born, might feel far-fetched. I've said this to people with a worthiness wound before, and their response is something along the lines of "That's a nice idea and I hear your words, but I just don't feel that. I don't even know what it means." And honestly, it's okay if the jury is out right now. It's okay if you think that everyone else in the world is worthy and you aren't. But I'd really like for us to explore and see if we can shake something up together and make it make more sense, okay?

How did you come to believe you are too fat, too emotional, or not good enough for love? Where did that story originate? Who put it there in the first place? And how did you come to believe you are unworthy? As with all our wounds, the answer is simpler than it may seem.

There is an origin story that convinces you that you are.

I'm Unworthy Because . . .

The more time I spend with people, the more I'm convinced that we might all have some type of worthiness wound. At the very minimum, maybe our worthiness gets questioned from time to time.

> Corinna wakes up before her boyfriend every morning, does her makeup, then gets back into bed so that when he wakes up, he thinks she's effortlessly beautiful.
> Christof is convinced that until he makes more money, he'll just be overlooked by the women he's attracted to.
> Ari believes their chronic illness will be too exhausting for a partner and that thus they will never marry.

These narratives, the stories these individuals tell themselves about themselves, reveal a worthiness wound.

Where did it begin, the story about how you came to believe that you were unworthy of love, of being chosen, of being wanted, of someone sticking around, or of being good enough? Do you remember the words or the explicit statements? Do you remember the actions? Do you remember what it felt like to learn that love was conditional? Or the story that abandonment left you with?

When I started working with Veronica, she was in her early fifties. She was single, had never been married, and didn't have any kids. She had been in therapy for decades, but she wasn't seeing much progress. She had worked on Wall Street for thirty years and spoke in harsh and abrasive tones. She had told me her vocal cords were exhausted from all the smoking and the shouting over the men she had had to do for decades.

She gave me a look, smiled, and said, "I'm not aggressive, I'm just tired. This place takes it outta ya. Anyway, I thought this therapy stuff was supposed to work. It's not working for me. You're my last shot."

This was how she began our first session.

"That's a lot of pressure." I smiled. "We better get to work, then."

Veronica wasn't ready to hear that it wasn't me who was her last shot, it was her, but she'd soon come to learn that in our sessions.

Veronica shared that she liked that therapy was a place where someone would listen to her. It felt good to vent and get it out. What she didn't like was that it seemed like nothing ever changed.

"I'm not getting a good ROI," she said.

Just so you know, ROI stands for return on investment. And I hear something along those lines from almost all my clients who work in the financial world. They talk about ROI and cost-benefit analysis and data points. (Don't forget the data points!)

Veronica felt she had spent a lot of money and time on therapy over the years, and the return she was getting was the same old outcome year after year. Her investment in therapy was not yielding the outcome she wanted.

"I want a partner. I'm clearly over the kids thing, but I really want to love and be loved."

With very little digging I learned that Veronica had never talked about her family with her previous therapists. I am all for different modalities and theories; in fact I'm a big believer that no one model will fit all. But—and this is a big but—I cannot for the life of me imagine therapy without prioritizing understanding the relationships in one's family system and the origin stories associated with them.

"Is it okay if we spend some time talking about your family?" I asked.

"Yeah, sure. Do your thing."

Since I was Veronica's last shot, she was ready and willing to go in whatever direction I took her. I started asking her about her family and found out right away that her mother had left them when Veronica was just five years old.

"Do you know why she left?" I asked.

"Yeah, she never really wanted children. My mom just wanted to live the good life. She didn't want any responsibilities; she didn't want to be held down or lose her freedom. She packed one bag and left on a Saturday morning like it was any other Saturday morning. Some woman pulled into the driveway and honked. She pulled my sister and me in close, got down to our height level, and said, 'I love you both so very much, but this isn't good for Mama.' She smiled and waved as her friend pulled out of the driveway and we never saw her again."

Veronica wasn't emotional at all when she shared this with me. She was caught in what I call *factual storytelling*. This is when you spill the details of what happened without any connection to the emotion attached to it or to the impact that it had or has on you. Factual storytelling is a type of invulnerability, a way of protecting yourself from what you believe is too much to feel and be present with.

Veronica had become a professional factual storyteller. She was entertaining and captivating when she spoke. She could make others feel something, but she wouldn't let herself feel *anything*.

Veronica had shared her story plenty of times with friends, colleagues, and new acquaintances she'd meet at bars. She'd just never shared it with her therapists. Why?

"They never asked." She shrugged.

And she was right. They hadn't. But Veronica hadn't offered it up, either. She was smart. She knew that this was a big piece of her story; she just didn't want to *go there*. At least not until now.

Veronica had followed me on Instagram for over a year and understood my framework. She knew she was signing up for diving into her family of origin, and she knew that this style of therapy wasn't limited to venting. We rolled up our sleeves and got to work together.

With her mother's departure, Veronica had been left with an origin story of unworthiness.

Sometimes a sense of worthiness is eradicated in a single moment, and other times it is slowly stripped away through a series of events or messages. In Veronica's case, her mother's abandonment had left her believing she was not a good enough daughter for her mother to stick around.

Like many who feel unworthy, Veronica was desperate to find someone who would prove her worthiness. But as much as she wanted partnership, it just wasn't happening for her. She'd start romantic relationships, and after a few months they'd end. Many things can contribute to a worthiness origin wound, and Veronica could check each one off. She didn't believe that people would stay. She believed that she wasn't good enough, valuable enough, or important enough for someone to want to be with her. She would choose men who were unavailable, or she'd choose men who were available but would find ways to push them away.

She told me how she'd task the available men with endless things.

The tester in me could see the tester in her. She'd have them drop off and pick up her dry cleaning, schedule the housecleaners, book her flights, and make sure the refrigerator was stocked for her. She treated them like an employee instead of a partner. But for a long time she couldn't see what the problem was.

Until we began doing origin healing work together, Veronica would test her partners in such significant ways that they would eventually walk away. She was on a sabotage mission, but she was blind to the fact. It was time for Veronica to see how her past was running the show and keeping her looped in unhealthy relationship patterns. It was time for Veronica to dig in and see what a significant impact her childhood had had on her.

So where did *your* worthiness wound come from? As the Swiss psychiatrist and psychoanalyst Carl Jung would say, "Until you make the unconscious conscious, it will direct your life and you will call it fate." You, too, must dig in and begin to see your childhood more clearly. As we'll see, parents who are unavailable, conditional in their love, or hypercritical contribute significantly to feelings of unworthiness. Did a parent or significant person in your life display any of these traits?

UNAVAILABILITY

A parent's unavailability has an impact on you. There's always a story behind someone's lack of availability, but having parents who were unavailable to you is painful, confusing, and lonely, and it often results in a worthiness wound. Home is where we want to be able to go for guidance, love, connection, and comfort. Of course, believing that we are worthy is ultimately an inside job, but when we are children, our worth is tied to how the adults in our life treat us, speak to us, and speak about us. Home is the first place we learn whether we matter or not, whether we are worthy or not, or whether we are deserving or not. Families of origin are critical in establishing and maintaining worthiness in children, and family relationships play a central role in shaping children's well-being over the course of their lives.

Unavailability can take the form of inconsistency. Or of absence. Or, in extreme cases, as with Veronica, of abandonment.

Inconsistency is one of the most common forms of unavailability. Think about parents who send mixed messages. One day they're your biggest cheerleader when it comes to helping you with your homework, and on other days they're critical of you for not being able to figure it out yourself. Or perhaps your parents knew supportive things to say when you were having big emotions and then, other times, told you to suck it up or deal with it on your own. Or parents who, when you made a mistake or did something upsetting to them, could talk to you about it in a kind and loving way, while at other times they were critical, mean, and punishing. As the research shows, if a parent, especially a mother, is inconsistent in praise, acknowledgment, and expressions of love, the child may suffer from a lack of self-esteem and be more vulnerable to depression.

You may have experienced inconsistency from a parent if:

- *You didn't know what version of your parent you would get.* The kind and loving parent or the highly critical one. The playful and lighthearted one or the angry and reactive one.

- *You couldn't predict your parents' reaction or what the consequences might be.* Sometimes they would be lenient; other times they would be extremely punitive.

- *You weren't sure how they'd communicate with you.* Your parents sometimes spoke to you with care and consideration and other times didn't care how their words would impact you.

- *You never knew their level of interest in your life.* Sometimes they had interest in your life and other times they didn't. Sometimes they had time or energy for you and other times didn't.

A significant amount of inconsistency can leave you feeling confused about whether you were valued or important to your parents, as well as leave you questioning your self-worth and adequacy.

Here I need to note that I'm *not* talking about a parent who missed a few soccer games out of the hundreds you had, or a parent who had to finish a work project at home from time to time but was otherwise a present and loving parent. What I am talking about is a level of inconsistency that was so disorienting and confusing that it created the conditions for you to question your worth.

Inconsistency isn't the only way parents make themselves unavailable. Sometimes parents remove themselves entirely and are physically or emotionally unavailable. Absent parents might be gone for months at a time due to work, have a mental health challenge that has them checked out of life and parenting, have started a new family and committed themselves to their new partner and the children they have together more than to you, or just not want to be bothered.

An absent parent, no matter the reason, can leave you questioning your worth. Sure, the reasons they are absent might give some context. But put yourself in a child's shoes for a moment. Most children aren't emotionally mature enough to understand the reasons surrounding the absence or the constraints of their parents. What they tend to do instead is take it personally, especially when no other alternative story makes sense to them.

In Veronica's case, unavailability happened through abandonment. Her mom left her father, sister, and her behind without any explanation other than it's "not good for Mama."

What's *not good for Mama*?

For Veronica, it meant that *she* wasn't.

A worthiness wound was beginning to take up space in her five-year-old body, and it was setting the foundation for a lifetime of questioning her worth.

"My sister and I cried for days after my mom left. Because she was my older sister by two years, I looked to her for an explanation. As if a seven-year-old would have any of the answers. She and I would talk and talk and talk. We'd look through Mom's stuff to see if we could find any hints, but there was nothing. We came to the conclusion together that it had to be us. Nothing else made sense. If being a mom wasn't good for her, then it was her children who were the problem. Right? I mean, really, try to disprove that."

After sitting with the pain she'd surfaced for a moment and acknowledging it, I said, "It must feel impossible to believe that you're deserving of lasting partnership that will stick around when your mom didn't."

This wasn't really a question; I already knew the answer.

Veronica knew the answer, too, but this was the first time someone had said this to her in such a direct way.

Can you look back at your childhood to see if your parents were unavailable to you in any way? And can you feel what it was like for you when this inconsistency, absence, or abandonment took place?

Let's try it together, shall we?

- The person who was unavailable to me growing up was _____.

- The type of unavailability I experienced was [inconsistency, absenteeism, abandonment] _____, and what I remember about that experience was _____.

You're doing beautiful work here. You're starting to lean into the process. Unavailability might not be all you remember. There are multiple way parents contribute to their child's unworthiness wound.

CONDITIONAL LOVE

I believe that love can be unconditional, while relationships need to have conditions. This is true for partnership, adult familial relationships, and friendship. But for children, unconditional love is particularly important, especially as they move through a new world of firsts. Unconditional love separates children from their behavior, and it communicates to them that mistakes are okay, that mess-ups are allowed, and that disappointment can happen without their love and worthiness being at stake.

Withholding love, communication, or forgiveness as a form of punishment can be one of the most gut-wrenching psychological and painful experiences a child can experience. My father used to do this often. If I was difficult (that is to say, behaving like a kid or a teenager) and he didn't like what was happening, he'd burst out in anger and then I would be given the silent treatment for days or even weeks at a time. This was a cruel form of punishment. I didn't know then what I know now. His reactivity was a result of his not being able to be with his own emotions or mine. He didn't know how to tolerate emotion, so he learned to react in this way. *This* was his way of communicating, of teaching me a lesson, and of using power and control to get his way. But I didn't like his way. And I also wasn't one to back down. I learned to be silent in return, matching him day by day, week by week. *Who would speak first?* I could play this game. But playing this game didn't change the fact that it was contributing to my belief that something bad would happen if I was difficult. Something bad *did* happen when I was difficult; love became conditional.

Just so we're clear, when I make the distinction between the kind of conditional love that results in a worthiness wound and the kind of unconditional love that children need, I am not talking about an absence of consequences. Rather, I'm talking about reinforcing consequences when it's necessary while also reassuring children that they're still loved. What I really needed him to say was some version of "I really don't like that you did that, and you won't be able to go spend time with your friends this weekend, but I love you and am happy to talk this through with you when you're ready."

I love you and I'm available. That's the reassurance. *I love you and you matter to me. I love you and I'm not going anywhere. I love you and you're safe. I love you and I forgive you. No matter what you do, the love isn't going to go anywhere, even if there must be consequences to your actions. I love you.*

I didn't need him to let me off the hook. I needed him to set a consequence and reassure me that his love was a constant. Yet his inconsistency created a worthiness wound around my behavior—I was being too difficult—that intersected with my belief concerning my worthiness. *Don't be difficult and you'll be okay. Be difficult and you risk relationships and love.*

My experience with my father taught me that if I behaved a certain way, I'd have access to love, connection, communication, and presence. He'd be happy to do things for me, cook me dinner, or help me with my homework. But if I crossed some invisible line, those things would be lost. Such behavior from him would continue into my early twenties. If I was a "good girl," he'd be happy to grab some items from the grocery store to help me out in a pinch or to pick me up from the train station as I made the commute from New Jersey to New York for work daily.

But the minute I said something he didn't like or that hurt his feelings, he would punish me. I'd get a call from him at ten P.M. saying that I'd have to find someone else to pick me up the next morning at six to take me to the train station. Yes, I had alternatives—I had a car and could have driven myself and parked; I could have called for a cab—but I didn't have much extra money back then and that wasn't even the point. The point was that he was punishing me. The point was that he was using withholding behavior to communicate something to me. I learned that if I behaved a certain way, it kept connection, presence, love, and ease alive; if I didn't behave that way, they would be gone. This taught me that I was worthy when I was easy and agreeable, and unworthy when I wasn't.

- What conditions were set around love in your family?
- What were the conditions you needed to meet in order to have connection or presence?
- What conditions did you need to meet to be respected and valued in your family?

Conditional love strips away a sense of respect and value for an individual. Critical commentary can be just as demoralizing, if not more so.

STATEMENTS OF HARM

For some, a worthiness origin wound is packaged very clearly with no room for misunderstanding. Rather than just making themselves unavailable or putting conditions on their love, some parents, to put it bluntly, say explicitly to their children that they are worthless. They tell them that they'll never amount to anything, that they were a mistake and should never have been born, or that they are useless and a pathetic excuse for a human. This is abusive. Full stop. These words are cutting, harmful, and deeply damaging. We'll discuss abuse later in another chapter, but it's important to acknowledge that a worthiness wound can come from someone telling us directly that we are in fact not worthy.

Sometimes this happens repeatedly, the damage done in a number of ways; sometimes it occurs in one outburst where the words can't be unheard. And sometimes it's through shame and judgment. The way our parents speak to us and the words they use tell us a lot about them . . . but when we're children, their words tell us the most about ourselves.

Veronica didn't feel the full weight of her father's criticism until after her mother left. It started with insidious comparisons to her sister, Carol. After her mother's abandonment, Veronica struggled in school and elsewhere. Her dad's reaction was to make angry, critical comments about how she needed to be more like her sister. He'd say, "Why can't you study harder like her?" Or "If you were more like Carol, my life would be much simpler."

His comments were really hurtful. Veronica *had* started acting out. But rather than reassuring her, her dad criticized her even more.

"Our mom had just abandoned us, and those comments put me over the edge. All he could say was 'Be more like your sister.' Be more like my sister and what? I'll love you more? Be more like my sister and I'll actually acknowledge that your mother left? Be more like my sister and your mom might return?" Veronica's voice broke. She closed her eyes and wept. In addition to the fact her mother had abandoned her, her father's statements of harm made her continue to question her worth. *I can't even get love from the parent who's still here.*

Not all statements of harm are explicitly cruel. Sometimes they are more subtle. Maya had a loving family who supported her, but her mother, who also struggled with body image issues, would constantly tell her that she should never get more than five pounds away from her ideal weight. "Don't let it get too out of control," her mother would say. She would follow this up with "But I love you despite the pounds."

Oof, that word *despite*. It cuts, doesn't it? Maya had always been at odds with her body. *If I don't lose the weight, no one will want me. If I don't lose the weight, no one will find me attractive. If I don't lose the weight, I'm not worthy of partnership.* These were the messages the subtle-not-so-subtle comments from her mother decades earlier left her with.

When you look back at your childhood, can you remember the

words that your parents spoke to you that left a lasting impact? Maybe they still say the same words today, like Maya's mom, who still comments about those extra pounds. Or maybe it was a comment that was spoken only once but stuck in your head forever. I'm reminded constantly how one cutting remark can set the tone and a narrative around worth for decades to come.

My client Trevor told me that he needs to be really good friends with someone before he dates them, because if they get to know him first, then his height won't be the reason they pass over him. This all stems from an offhand remark made by a girl he had a crush on in fifth grade. At a party she said, "You'd be cute if you were just taller." And there it was. A remark that left him questioning his worth for a very long time.

I know it's not fun to think back on hurtful and critical comments. But words come with us and it's important that we acknowledge the impact they have.

- The person whose words were most hurtful growing up was _____.

Again, you might notice sensations in your body that start to shift as you name the above. It's just information, so it's okay to make some space for it.

- The words hurt because _____.

Do you remember that childhood rhyme "Sticks and stones may break my bones, but words will never hurt me"? Yeah, it's BS. They sold us a crock of lies packaged as resiliency. The words hurt. They're allowed to hurt. Let yourself acknowledge that they hurt.

To explore the origins of your worthiness wound is no small undertaking. Identifying how you came to believe you are unworthy can be deeply emotional. Maybe you recognized something for the first time, or maybe you were reminded of something you already knew. Either way, there's a wound there that you likely found a way to cope with.

Coping with the Worthiness Wound

There are many possible ways children will respond if their worthiness is being threatened or in question. Some will become perfectionists. Others will aim to please or will become as useful as possible to show that they have something valuable to offer. Some will focus on performance and achievement, believing that if they do well, they'll be worthy of attention, validation, and celebration. They'll do everything in their power to make their parents happy, hoping that a happy parent will equate to being a worthy child.

Some will stay on this path eternally, well after they leave their family of origin. They'll continue to present themselves as perfect, be useful to those around them, perform, and please, all with the hope of being convinced that they are deserving of good things, of love, attention, connection, and intimacy. Others might try those things but eventually acquiesce to accepting that they are unworthy.

At that event I hosted years ago, the room was filled with people who had a worthiness wound. But that room of people is *every* room of people. It's your partner and it's you. It's your friends, your coworkers, your parents, and your boss. You don't have to look far to find someone with a worthiness wound, someone who doesn't feel good enough.

If you were a child who tried to be perfect, become useful, perform and achieve, or please, I want you to know that I see how hard you tried. *Of course* you did those things. *Of course* you gave it what you had. You were doing everything in your power to secure a sense of worthiness for youself. You were working overtime to ensure that you felt deserving. What beautiful attempts at creating safety and a confident path forward for yourself. And maybe you can also acknowledge these attempts of yours at securing a sense of worthiness, too.

Hand on heart. Let's try it. Can you acknowledge how hard you worked at protecting yourself? Can you offer gratitude for what you have accomplished?

"Thank you for _____. I appreciate how hard you worked because _____."

It's important that you shift from self-criticism to self-gratitude. But it usually isn't that simple. Something more might need to shift, or your old ways may no longer serve you in the ways they once did. But how we learned to operate and survive was once of immense value and importance to us, so we ought to acknowledge it with respect, gratitude, and admiration if we can make some space for it.

Healing the Worthiness Wound

Shifting and changing is the work we must do, but it isn't always easy. For a long time, Veronica couldn't see her part in her unhappy relationships. The blame was always on others. Partners didn't care enough, didn't try hard enough, and didn't love her enough. We needed to shift her from her victim mentality so that she could see how she was participating. Without this, she'd continue to re-create these dynamics and keep blaming everyone else.

As my relationship with Veronica developed and more trust was established, I was able to help her take an even closer look at her worthiness wound. "I think you're making it really hard for people to choose you, Veronica." I said it with tenderness, as I knew this might be hard to hear. "People don't want to be your help. They want to be your partner. They want to get to know you. They don't want to be given an endless number of tasks by you."

Veronica was beginning to see how she was pushing people away. She made it nearly impossible for people to get to know her, because if they weren't jumping through all her hoops, she'd react strongly. "Why can't you just help me? Am I not important enough for you to prioritize this? Am I not valuable enough in your life for you to just do the things I ask you to?" she'd ask her partners.

Veronica was unconditionally worthy, and so are you. You are worthy of love, connection, presence, attention, safety, and beyond. You are worthy of it. But you also can't just act however you want and believe that a relationship will thrive anyway. As we journeyed into Veronica's origin stories, she was able to see how her worthiness wound was sabotaging her relationships. She was learning that she couldn't push people away and expect them to stay. She needed to stop testing and learn to create some boundaries and establish some guidelines. Otherwise she'd continue to lose relationships and prove her story of unworthiness true.

Veronica's healing required her to be in relationship with her victim part. She'd have to set boundaries with it and continue to strengthen the belief that she was worthy. She *could* have a successful relationship, as long as she brought awareness to the part of herself that kept telling her that she couldn't. Instead of choosing unavailable men or finding ways to avoid connection and intimacy with those who were available, Veronica would steadily begin to open herself up to connection. When she'd feel the urge to give her partner some new chore or throw down a gauntlet for him to take up, she'd remind herself that this was a tactic her worthiness wound would use to prove a story she no longer wanted to prove. Veronica worked hard at this. But *this* work was rewarding work. *This* work had a phenomenal ROI.

Origin Healing Practice: The Steps

I'm going to walk you through four steps that I believe are vital in your healing journey. I call this our Origin Healing Practice. This framework builds off the endless therapeutic wisdom about how change happens, but this is what has worked for me and for many of my clients. The steps are to *name* the wound, to *witness* and honor it, to *grieve* the loss of your authentic self, and finally, as the wound begins to heal, to *pivot* to new behaviors and choices.

Once I've explained the four steps in detail, there will be an opportunity for you to do the Origin Healing Practice yourself. We will come back to this four-step practice for each wound in part 2, and you'll dive into the ones that resonate most for you. How you move through this is nuanced and personal, and there's no one "right" way to do it. The practice won't necessarily be easy at first. Do what you can. You'll come back to this many times over. You might find yourself experiencing stronger feelings than you usually do. You might be processing your memories and emotions in a more intentional way than you ever have before. Stick with it. If you engage in the Origin Healing Practice, you will see the many opportunities for change, growth, and healing.

NAME WHAT WAS

If you can't acknowledge the wound, it's pretty hard to heal it. And if you acknowledge it incorrectly, you're likely to find yourself on the wrong healing path. Someone else's story that's similar to yours may have left them with an origin wound but might not leave you with the same one. I know, I know, this is where it can get tricky, but it's why spending time with your story, noticing the details, and identifying what was wounding for you will set you on *your* healing path. That's why I always say, "Call it exactly what it is—no more, no less." This is a bold first step. One that requires you to connect to bravery as you lean toward naming what was, as it was.

You might remember Natasha from the first chapter, and how hard it was for her to name her father's infidelity—and just as challenging, the subtle expectation that she would participate in the betrayal. Or Veronica, who in her previous attempts at therapy had managed never to speak about her family at all in order to conceal a worthiness wound. Maybe the idea of naming your wound—perhaps acknowledging its origin in your parents' or caretaker's unavailability, conditional love, or statements of harm—feels risky to you, too. This stage puts you face-to-face with the things that had an impact on you and asks you to be honest about them without minimizing, maximizing, invalidating, or distorting the story in any way. It's important to slow down and name what once was. If you don't confront the past, the unidentified may run the show. And I can promise you, it will.

CAN I GET A WITNESS?

To be witnessed is one of the most profound experiences of a lifetime. Let's define what that means in this therapeutic context, though. To be *witnessed* means that you (yes, you can witness your own story) or someone else honors your story by bearing witness to it—to your pain, and to the things that impact or have impacted you. You are heard; you are seen; you are acknowledged.

Having your experience witnessed can change the trajectory of your life, quite literally. This simple acknowledgment can help you unhook from a pattern you're trying to break free from. Don't underestimate the power of it. This act of witnessing means to be present to what was or is by seeing it, feeling it, connecting to it, and experiencing it firsthand (or as if it were firsthand).

The power of being deeply seen is sometimes all it takes for a pattern to release its grip.

I remember the first time I felt truly witnessed by my now husband. (This step makes me emotional to even write about.) I was having a phone conversation with a family member who was committed to defending herself over hearing what I was sharing. This was a dynamic that had played out between us over and over again across decades, and I felt exhausted by it. My wounded part kept trying to get the other person to hear me, to understand my hurt, to take ownership for her part in it. My attempts were failing miserably, and every time I failed, I felt more hurt.

This evening Connor was at home, and I happened to have the phone on speaker during the tense and frustrating conversation. He sat there, listening to the exchange. The conversation went as it always did, but what happened next was so healing that it released something within me.

I got off the phone and Connor and I connected. He explained to me what he had listened to and heard. And unbelievably, his experience of it was *my* experience of it. He heard the same things I did in the conversation, and he validated my feelings and frustrations. Not only was he witnessing me in that moment, but he was also witnessing *every version* of me prior. I'd had the same argument again and again with this family member, going back decades. My inner child felt as seen, as did the adult me.

Somehow, though nothing had changed in the dynamic between me and my family member, I didn't feel alone anymore. I no longer needed them to "get it" and understand my point of view; it was enough for someone else to. This one moment disengaged me from a decades-long unhealthy pattern.

Just take that in for a moment. Witnessing does not need to be person dependent. Of course, we may desire for a particular person to hear us, but what I have found personally and professionally to be true is that to be witnessed well by *anyone* can change the course.

Sometimes the original person who contributed to the wounding is able to hear your truth. Sometimes this happens with a partner. Sometimes this happens with a friend. Sometimes you slow down enough to do it for yourself. And, as is the case at all of the retreats I've ever hosted, it happens with strangers. Brave souls who come together for a few days; individuals who have never met one another before and may never spend another day together outside of the retreat setting, who bear witness to one another and participate in a stage of healing that is life altering.

The moments when I find myself getting hooked back into the pattern are when I know it's time to be witnessed again. It isn't always one and done; in fact, it rarely is. In these moments of reactivation I can turn to my partner, to dear friends who understand, or to my own self.

MAKE SPACE FOR GRIEF

When most of us think about grief, we think about it in relation to losing someone we love. In our family of origin work together, the process of grieving is in response to you losing a part of *yourself*— losing who you were, your authentic self *before* the wounds, pain, and trauma took place. And that's not all you have to grieve. Many of us must also release the ways we have learned to cope that have disconnected us further from ourselves, ways that we've treated ourselves that are particularly painful to acknowledge. Maybe you coped with the pain by treating your body poorly. Maybe you coped with the wounds by engaging in sexual relationships with people you didn't want to be intimate with. Or maybe you coped by becoming critical of yourself, badgering yourself repeatedly. You'll work on grieving, and thus letting go of, those maladaptive coping strategies as well.

Both witnessing and grieving can be emotional processes. When you're properly witnessed, either by yourself or by another, you experience a release. It's like a valve opens, and what has been closed off suddenly begins to flow. You shift from protection mode to something much more open and kinetic.

When the valve is closed, we tend to brace ourselves. There's a tension present in the body. It's hard to feel our emotions fully when that's the case, and the emotion is either denied or repressed.

Grieving in this context is being present to *all* of the feelings that show up once you've been witnessed. Once the valve opens, allow yourself to be with it and feel it. I bet you can already anticipate it—once you make space for those feelings, they are going to come rushing in! That's normal and expected. There is no right way, no proper speed at which you ought to move through these feelings as you confront your grief. Just know that you will eventually need to feel your way through. You can't avoid your way through, deny your way through, or repress your way through. That's what got you here in the first place. *You have to feel your feels, my friend.*

Remember: What was taken from you is not lost forever. You can claim back your worth, belonging, prioritization, safety, and trust. You can claim back your sense of worth, your feelings of playfulness, ease, and joy.

PIVOT TO A NEW PATH

The athlete in me has always felt that this word properly depicts this step. The pivot is a quick change in direction. If you pivot well on the field or on the court, your opponent shouldn't see it coming. Your unhealthy patterns, like a good defense, anticipate your next step.

Your job is to change it up on them. Patterns thrive on your consistency, so if you want to modify an unhealthy pattern, you will need to become inconsistent, at least until you can become consistent with something that is much healthier and more aligned to you.

This work requires your awareness. This is where you begin to choose how you lead yourself to a new outcome. After Connor had witnessed me, there were plenty of times when I needed to witness myself and spend a lot of time grieving. This release, as I mentioned before, led me to realize that I didn't need to engage with the family member in the same way anymore. This realization was not the pivot itself; the pivot was every time I didn't engage. The pivot happened in every moment that the old pattern would try to play itself out and I wouldn't engage.

Pivoting is a recommitment to the self. It says, *I see you AND I honor you.* The latter is possible because enough witnessing and grieving have taken place to allow it. It's very hard to pivot without that. That's why you can mean well, put your head down, commit to your goals, make promises to yourself over and over again, and still find yourself doing the same dance with the same or different people. If you're having trouble changing something that you want to transform, it means you haven't witnessed and grieved enough. Your system won't allow you to move on from the pain without first identifying it, witnessing it, and feeling it. This is not meant to be torture. Instead, it's designed to honor your pain and wounds.

I can tell you with great certainty that there is much liberation and freedom once you can call the thing the thing. I am reminded of one of my favorite quotes from Iyanla Vanzant: "When you can look a thing dead in the eye, acknowledge that it exists, call it exactly what it is, and decide what role it will take in your life then, my Beloved, you have taken the first step toward your freedom." You're doing it, friend. You're taking that first step toward your freedom.

Getting Started

If you're ready to take this healing practice a bit further, I'd recommend carving out some time and privacy for yourself. Again, this exercise is directed to those with a worthiness wound. If this isn't you, feel free to skip ahead to the next chapter to work through the identification process for the belonging wound. Each chapter in part 2 has a specific Origin Healing Practice associated with it, so you can do whichever ones apply to the wounds you've identified as yours. Go to www.viennapharaon.com/audio to listen to a guided Origin Healing Practice for each of the five origin wounds.

The process of healing is a very sacred experience. It can transport us. I generally encourage getting comfortable either by putting pillows down and wrapping yourself in a blanket or sitting on a meditation cushion and lighting a candle. Yes, you're setting the mood to heal.

Whatever feels safest for you is what you can do. I like to close my eyes so I can be fully present. That works for me, but some people prefer to keep their eyes open, as it helps them feel safe. They know no one is in their space, and they can see what's happening around them. There is no right or wrong way to do this, just your own way. This also might be something you prefer to do with your therapist. Take a look and see. If you're moving through trauma, you must take good care. Having someone who can guide you, support you, and help create a safe space for you while you do this work is necessary.

Let's begin:

NAMING Bring into focus the first moment you remember questioning your worth. Be gentle in this space. See if you can bring into focus the details of that first time.

Where were you? Who was there? How old were you? What were you wearing? Was it something someone else said that made you question your worthiness? Notice as many details as possible.

WITNESSING Become more focused on yourself, on the younger version of you that you're witnessing (not the you in this moment doing the exercise). And as if you were watching yourself on a video, I want you to notice the feelings you were experiencing in that former moment. When Veronica did this exercise, she watched her five-year-old self be told by her mother that her mother was going to leave. She watched herself watch her mom get into that car and drive off. Veronica was watching her younger self experience that moment and started to feel for that little girl, who with that event began to question her worth.

GRIEVING You might start to feel emotion here. Can you let it come? You might be attuned to what it must have been like for you all those years earlier. Your heart might break for your younger self who had to endure an abandonment or process statements of harm. Your heart might break for your younger self who began living inauthentically to please others or receive love. Feel for your younger self and notice what you want to offer them in this moment. Do you want to hug her? Do you want to tell him that you're so sorry he ever had to go through that? Do you want to pick them up and tell them it's going to be okay? What are you feeling compelled to do? And just notice that. Let the emotion come.

Be here for as long or as little feels comfortable to you. If your eyes are closed, take some time before you enter back into the room. Keep your eyes closed and bring some movement back into your fingertips, into your toes. Maybe stretch your neck. Maybe put your hands on your heart or your belly. Maybe bring awareness back into your breath. Think about what you'll see when you open your eyes. Can you remember where you are? And ever so slowly, flutter your eyes open. Take your time here.

What a big step you've just taken. Grieving isn't a one-time thing. You may need to revisit this exercise again and again. When I get intentional with my grieving, I tend to come into this over and over. I'll pick up new details, notice something new about my six- or nine-year-old self. It feels similar and new every time I spend time here. And so I offer that to you. As many times as you need, as you want. You may do this every day for a week. Or you might do it once and come back next year or in five years. I am so proud of you.

PIVOTING Can you think about the way your worthiness wound plays out today? In what relationships is it apparent to you? Do you please or perform, or do you hide or avoid to protect yourself from not feeling worthy? And if you could just take a moment, can you consider what would be different if you actually felt and knew you were worthy? In what way might you stop performing if you knew you were worthy of love? In what way would you stop hiding yourself if you felt valued and valuable? Pivoting requires you to get into the habit of slowing down, taking a moment, and getting clear on your next step.

Can you try finishing this sentence? *If I believed I was worthy, one way I would act differently is _____.* If you stopped doing that in the relationship you feel unworthy in, what would change? For this week I'd like you to see if you can just notice when there would be an opportunity to replace an old way with a new way. Just notice. There's nothing more you need to do now.

Whew. That's some serious work you've just done. Notice any tenderness or rawness you might be experiencing and take good care of yourself. Worthiness doesn't get established overnight. This, as is the case with all your origin healing work, will be a recommitment to the self over and over again. I see the work you're doing, and I can't wait to keep walking alongside you.

4

I WANT TO BELONG

Every child, every human, craves to be a part of something. We want to be ourselves and yet be part of that which is greater than ourselves. We want to belong.

When a family or group doesn't ask us to betray our authenticity, we feel honored and safe. A beautiful sense of belonging can emerge. To be part of something is important and deeply valuable.

Unfortunately, many families and groups have ways of being in which they consciously or unconsciously expect you to mold yourself to fit their expectations and maintain their ways. Too often individuals feel like they must sacrifice who they are to be part of a group, even to belong to their families. If only belonging was just given, instead of needing to be earned. But unfortunately, what we wish for doesn't always come, sometimes not ever and sometimes not easily. And children made to feel like outsiders will most likely become adults who still feel like they don't belong.

Origins of the Belonging Wound

"Why are there no other gay men in this city who want to settle down and just be normal???"

The door to my office wasn't even closed yet when a clearly frustrated Neil entered, fell into the sofa, and threw his head back. Neil was thirty-two and had started therapy with me about a month earlier after moving to New York from West Virginia a few months prior.

"What does *normal* mean?" I asked.

"Ugh, you know what I mean. A man who doesn't need to go out and party all the time. A man who wants monogamy. Wants to have nights in. Wants to commit. A man who doesn't need to make up for all the years we all lost being closeted."

Neil had just had another night out where he had partied hard. Prior to moving to New York, Neil had never done drugs and drank only occasionally. Now he felt out of control, and he came to me to figure out what was going on.

"Did you feel pressured by the people at the party?" I asked.

"No, not at all. That's what's crazy. There's literally no pressure, and yet here I am saying yes to something I don't want just because I'm being offered it and everyone around me is doing it."

I asked Neil if he thought that his new pattern of drug use was an attempt to fit in and ultimately belong.

He shrugged and started to reflect. "That's an interesting thought," he said.

Neil had dreamed of finding in New York City what he'd struggled to find back home: a community that made him feel normal. But it wasn't long before he realized that even within *his* community, the gay community, he still felt like an outsider. Neil wanted commitment, a life with someone else who shared similar values. But he was having trouble meeting men who wanted something more than a hookup. He was frustrated, but he didn't realize how affected he was until we started discussing it.

Neil had grown up smack-dab in the middle of two older brothers and two younger sisters. "I was the odd one out," he told me. "I wasn't into sports like my brothers, and I was always disappointing my dad. I wasn't the son that he expected or wanted. I knew that. And my mom and my sisters formed a girls' club where I wasn't welcome either."

Neil's parents were very religious, and everyone in their small hometown knew everyone's business. Neil had to get good at hiding anything he didn't want out in the open. And Neil was good at hiding that he was gay. He had hidden it from his family for fourteen years, and much longer from the hometown community. For years, Neil went to great lengths to fit in with his family. He tried the sports his dad wanted him to (even though he secretly hated them all), and he made a point of always talking about the girls he had crushes on. Neil played the part of the straight guy for a long time, but it didn't change the fact that he never felt like he fitted in.

When he did choose to share his sexuality with his parents, they didn't respond well. His worst nightmare came true. Not only were they not accepting, but they were judgmental and consumed by their own fears and insecurities.

When a family encounters differences, it can respond in a number of ways. Because Neil's parents had strong beliefs about sexuality, hearing that Neil was gay essentially caused a program overload for them. They believed that being gay is wrong, bad—a sin. And to have a son who was gay meant that they had failed as parents. They were so afraid of being judged by the rest of the community, they wound up passing that judgment on to Neil.

The night he told his parents, he overheard them speaking. "I remember my mom crying that night. I sat outside their bedroom door and listened to them talk about me. She told my dad that I was ruining her life. I cried every night for months because I couldn't understand why me being gay would ruin *her* life."

Everything changed and nothing changed. What persisted was Neil's lack of belonging. His parents started ignoring him around the home and would speak to him only about schedules and logistics. His siblings followed suit. His mother made it explicitly clear that while he was living under her roof, he was not to tell another soul about this. No one in their community could know. It didn't matter whether he was closeted or out, there was no way for him to fit in with his family.

He understood his news had shocked his parents. "They're from the South and they're very religious. I know this just doesn't compute for them, but I never thought they would treat me so differently. I thought they'd be upset but get over it and love me anyway." Intellectually, he understood his parents' struggle with it, but his heart ached. How could parents turn their backs on their child, making him a complete outsider?

We are all born unique. In a healthy environment, we're taught to embrace and celebrate the fact that every individual is different. We can be ourselves and be part of the group.

But sometimes the system of which we are a part doesn't accept those inherent differences. Furthermore, some parents don't know how to handle their child's divergence from the family. Which usually means that, at least early on, the child will have to cede to the parent.

As a kid, you don't have a say in the beliefs you are given. Fitting in is the golden ticket. The threat of not belonging usually pushes people into a corner, where they're asked to choose either the group or themselves. To choose oneself is too risky for a child. We'd much rather belong to the group. External belonging offers acceptance, validation, and pleasure, even when it's an illusion. No wonder most of us just try to fit in at first.

At some point, though, the differences likely began to chafe. Perhaps you pushed back against conformity early in life. Or you grew up to challenge your parents' beliefs. Or you drifted apart much later, when you were already an adult. Perhaps you even found a group or place to live, as did Neil, that supported your difference and liberated you to assert who you really were. Whether the distancing from the family's beliefs and lifestyles begins early on or much later in life, if a parent's capacity for embracing difference is limited, the result will be a child who believes that he is disapproved of. If a parent or group can't or doesn't leave enough space for alternative ways of being, the child will feel that rejection of his essence. Your way now conflicts with their way, and when parents are unable to reconcile the two, the result is active conflict and a belonging wound.

IGNORING AND AVOIDANCE

A family's response to a child's difference is sometimes to simply avoid it. Adults convince themselves that if they just look the other way and disregard something, it will cease to exist—or at the very minimum, they won't need to deal with it. Sometimes the adults do this to protect themselves, and sometimes they do it because they think they're protecting their child.

But as I always say, you can't avoid your way toward healing. And you also can't avoid your way toward acceptance and reconciliation. When a family responds to your differences by ignoring and avoiding you, it's no wonder a belonging wound can emerge.

I met Trish back in 2015, but her story has stayed with me. Trish had cerebral palsy (CP). It's a condition she was born with that affects her movement, muscle tone, and posture. Trish walked with a limp and had to work much harder than a fully able person would to sit down and stand up. Yet Trish's family never discussed her cerebral palsy. "Anytime I asked them what was wrong with me, they would say that nothing was. They wanted me to be normal so badly that they just pretended like nothing was wrong. They ignored my CP entirely."

This was greatly destabilizing for Trish. She *knew* something was different, but her family wouldn't acknowledge it. People at school would make fun of her daily, but when she would come home and try to get her questions answered, she was told that the kids were "just being mean" and that there was nothing wrong. Trish's parents attempt to protect Trish and themselves only created more destabilization and confusion. Andrew Solomon, a professor of clinical medical psychology and the author of the *New York Times* bestselling book *Far from the Tree,* talks about what he calls *horizontals,* the traits in a child that are foreign to the parent, like a physical disability, and how these horizontals are often treated as flaws, things that need fixing instead of acceptance and nurture.

Trish already felt different because of her cerebral palsy, and though her family didn't intend her any harm, their avoidance of her differences rather than an honoring of them exacerbated the wound in significant ways. Trish needed her parents to find a way to bridge the gap, to find a way to face whatever fears and doubts this activated for them. She needed them to be on her team, committed to finding the best path forward. "It was hard enough to have a different body, but having parents who can't even acknowledge it and your pain when you're literally begging them to was so damaging. It really messed with me for a long time, and I'm still trying to reconcile it," she said.

If you've ever had your reality denied, ignored, or avoided, you know how easy it can be to begin to question your own experience and your truth. Over time this can strip away your self-trust and leave you with little certainty and confidence. From that weakened position, you'll likely change yourself to fit in or accept yourself as an outsider.

In what way were you different from your family? In what way were you different from the world around you? Did your parents or anyone in your family system avoid or ignore your difference? In what way?

Let's try a bit of work together, okay?

- My difference was _____.
- The person/people who avoided and ignored my difference the most was _____.
- What would have been different if they could have acknowledged it is _____.

CONTROL

In contrast to other ways of dealing with difference, avoidance can seem like a benign strategy. For parents struggling with a child's difference that they don't have the capacity to accept, the fallback is often to try and exert control. Afraid of having their own beliefs and ways questioned or challenged, they preemptively limit what's perceived as acceptable behavior and what isn't. That way they never have to risk being wrong. It is far easier to tell another person *how* to be so that they themselves can stay the same than it is to create space for another to be and let that evolve and expand their own lives and perspective.

Carl grew up as a navy brat. He and his family were constantly moving. Carl was the oldest of three and was Mom's little helper when Dad was abroad. When Carl's father was home, he was extremely controlling. The children had to wake up to an alarm their father set, make their beds military style, and then do drills for hours before going to school. Carl's father had a way of being, believing, and doing. And he expected all his children to follow his way.

Carl hated participating in this early morning schedule. "We didn't sign up for the military. *He* did," Carl told me. Carl was wired differently from his siblings and would quietly beg and plead with his mom to talk to his father. She never did. "I went along with it all, but I was miserable" he told me during one session.

I asked Carl whether he felt like he could ever be honest with his dad about how he felt.

"He'd tell me what I wanted didn't matter and to essentially man up."

Many families have their own set of rules and expectations. And often very early on we learn what it means to be a part of our family and what's required of us. We might be taught about what religion we will practice, what etiquette is expected of us, how we need to look and dress, what life choices are acceptable, and whom we are allowed to like and love. Whether it's explicitly stated or not, the message sometimes becomes overpowering: *Operate as we operate, and you will belong; operate differently and you risk being allowed to be a part of us.* And it's when our family's expectations turn this controlling that a belonging wound can easily form.

Control doesn't just affect the child. It is often the parents' way of avoiding the risk of having to stand face-to-face with their own guilt, shame, or embarrassment. Control is an attempt at safety. Control keeps the people doing the controlling from facing their own fear that they themselves are not worthy, lovable, or good enough. *If I can choose for you, make you, get you to, or convince you that . . . then I can safely avoid my own fears. If I can get you to submit to me, then I don't have to ever surrender.* This is one of the greatest illusions for the person doing the controlling.

Controlling habits are also something that gets passed down through generations. Carl shared that his grandfather had been even more controlling than his father. As we discussed the origin of Carl's father's treatment of Carl in the treatment by *his* father, I could see Carl creating some space for understanding. He began to realize that his dad grew up being controlled and in pain and was just passing this down.

But understanding didn't change Carl's reality, and it won't change yours. It might offer some context, but it doesn't change the effect that control has on you. If you were controlled growing up, you likely struggled to feel like a central, valued, and respected part of the family.

Control has a tight grip. Its hold is suffocating and it works tirelessly to wring the difference out of you. This is a terrible experience to have, and it's no wonder that you eventually yield to the iron fist, go to war with it, or find some other creative way to be released.

Within the context of your difference with your family system, was there anyone who responded to it with control? Let's take a moment here to reestablish your difference. Can you name it?

- My difference was _____.

From here let's explore just a bit more:

- The person [people] who responded to that difference with control was _____.
- How they controlled me was _____.
- What stands out to me most about how the control made me feel was _____.

INTOLERANCE AND SHAME

Intolerance is the inability or unwillingness to accept views, beliefs, or a lifestyle that differs from one's own. Generally speaking, parents want what's best for their children. They want them to succeed, to be healthy, and to be loved and belong. But when intolerance rears its head, a family confronted by something new and different can close off entirely.

For Neil, it meant having parents who struggled to maintain their relationship with him for many years because accepting his sexuality would mean discarding their long-held beliefs. In order to accept and love their gay son, his parents would have had to update their rigid beliefs around sexuality, which in turn would challenge their core religious and political beliefs.

Intolerance might also look like parents who can't accept your loving someone who belongs to a faith other than the one you grew up with. Or maybe it's parents who don't accept the ways in which your political, religious, or racial views differ from theirs, and who find ways to ostracize you because of the differences.

When family members hold beliefs that allow for very little deviation or tolerance, they often resort to shaming or ejecting an individual who can't or doesn't conform. This has almost nothing to do with you and almost everything to do with them. Your differences reflect something back to them, often shedding a light on their own insecurities, doubts, and shame. When ignored, these dynamics are corrosive, to the individual as well as to the relationship.

Shame is arguably the most destructive response to difference. It will have you convinced that you are so deeply flawed that you can't be loved. It's awful enough when you shame yourself, but when you are shamed by others—especially the important people you look to for love, guidance, nurturing, and protection—it can be debilitating.

When I met Bri, her inner critic was vicious. The inner critic is what therapists call the self-critical voice inside your head. It usually has a lot to say, much of it unkind. But I've always said that the inner critic has an origin story, too—one that didn't start with your being unkind to yourself. That critic learned its criticism from somewhere, and Bri learned shame from her mother.

Bri grew up in an evangelical Christian household after her parents' divorce. Her mom had come to religion during some of her darkest days, but the way in which she practiced religion was severe. And Bri's ways, ordinary behavior typical of most adolescents, were unacceptable to her mother. When Bri bought her first thong, her mom had a meltdown. "She started crying and told me I was going to hell. I knew something was off even back then, but I absorbed the things she said as truth. I thought I was bad. Everything I did was shamed. Having a boyfriend, going to prom, dressing a certain way all elicited talk about how I was 'taking Satan's path.' It was crazy."

The incessant shaming left Bri feeling like she didn't belong. She didn't feel like she was doing anything wrong, but the feedback she was being given by one of the most important people in her life was telling her she was. For years Bri tried to live in such a way that her mother could accept. But eventually she accepted that she just couldn't please her.

Because there was no room for her to find her way without shame growing up, Bri internalized that shame and continued to struggle as an adult. When you're constantly judging, criticizing, and shaming *yourself*, you have no way to step into authenticity, to belong.

How were your differences shamed or judged? And can you think about how that shame and judgment have contributed to creating your self-critical voice? You might know your inner critic already, but can you identify its origin story? If you accept that your inner critic didn't start with your being unkind to yourself, can you figure out where it did start?

- The thing I hear most often from my inner critic is
  _____.
- My inner critic's origin story is _____.

IMPACT OF SOCIETAL SYSTEMS

More than ever before, we dread disagreeing with friends and strangers alike due to the increase in incivility. We are a much more polarized society than we've ever been before. People are living in fear of being canceled or living in fear of being exiled if their beliefs differ from those of their neighbor. It has become easier to conform and comply than it is to honor your authenticity.

Not all wounds start with your family of origin, and not every wound must happen early in your life. So when it comes to belonging wounds, it's especially important to honor the impact and pressure that society, marketing, community, and systems at large have on us all.

Everywhere you look, marketing preys and benefits off your insecurities. It takes advantage of our very natural fears of being different. Social media tools that create the "perfect" image distort reality and will have you comparing yourself to the "better" lives of everyone else. Because of FOMO (fear of missing out), we don't want to be the *only one* who doesn't have the experience that everyone else is going to have. Beauty standards in America have long validated the European beauty standard that emphasizes being fair-skinned, slim, and tall. And until recently, in television shows, movies, commercials, and magazines, there was little representation of different cultures, skin tones, a spectrum of sexuality, or so-called nontraditional romantic relationships, leaving millions of children and adults alike struggling to find themselves in *any* of the characters, relationships, or careers they see presented again and again.

No one wants to be othered. No one wants to feel left out. And no one wants to feel like an outsider. And yet this is what so many individuals experience. It's a lonely place to feel this way at home, at school, or in your community. That's why so many people will move toward what they believe will help them belong.

Code-switching is where a person learns to dial up or down an accent or a dialect, or change their behavior and appearance in order to fit in. This is common in groups when nonwhite individuals feel pressure to be "more white" or mainstream—like a Black or Brown child learning how to exist in a predominantly white community or school. Or someone who's gay presenting heteronormatively. Or someone who is nonbinary existing in binary systems. Or a child who goes to a private school on a full financial scholarship and attempts to hide the significant class difference.

When I met Vanessa, she seemed relieved to be in touch. She was trying to move forward from a bad breakup, but being a newly single parent while simultaneously processing and grieving the ending of a relationship was a nightmare for her. She felt embarrassed and ashamed and was dodging the "I told you so" commentary from friends and family about her ex, an athlete who was much younger than her.

"I know, I know," she let out, anticipating some judgment on my part about the age difference, but instead revealing her own.

Vanessa was an only child. Her father, who had passed away when she was younger, was Black, and her mother was white. Vanessa had grown up in an all-white community and gone to an all-white school. She had a lot of friends and enjoyed her childhood, but it was clear that in order for her to fit in, she felt she needed to be whiter. This meant dressing a certain way, doing her hair a certain way, and speaking a certain way. From elementary school through high school and college, she emphasized her whiteness to belong. Vanessa's Blackness, on the other hand, had to be toned down and at times even erased. Dr. Walker S. Carlos Poston proposes a theory of biracial identity development, describing how biracial or multiracial individuals feel pressure to choose one racial or ethnic group identity over the other. He maintains that this choice is heavily influenced by the relative status of the group, parental influences, cultural knowledge, and appearance. Vanessa's father was the one who taught her about Black history and mirrored back to her a part of herself that she couldn't find in any other family member. After he passed, she felt even more distant from her Black heritage. Only later would she come to understand the significance of this major loss in her life.

Vanessa was on a journey to belong, but what she kept finding was a new place where she didn't fit, from her skin color to being unmarried and a mom to not looking like the girlfriends and wives of most players in the league when she and her ex were together. Noting her own athletic build, she described the other girlfriends and wives as curvy, saying that their attire and hair and makeup just "wasn't her." Her self-descriptions always reinforced her outsider status. From her now all-white family to her friends to her new white neighborhood that was close to her mother, she was drowning in her otherness.

When Vanessa moved to New York City, she started to see herself in other people. Others looked like her and she looked like others. It was a breath of fresh air, and she had a sense of renewed optimism that maybe at last she could find her people. But her friends still made comments that positioned her on the outside: that she wasn't Black enough, even too light-skinned "for a mixed girl."

These comments caused her great pain and reinforced her belonging wound. Vanessa grew up in systems where her differences were obvious, but were rarely acknowledged or honored. When something goes unacknowledged, you move toward what gets acknowledgment. For Vanessa that meant being whiter. And when she finally began to allow more of her whole self to come forward, she *still* struggled to fully fit in.

Without question, you've been impacted by societal systems. They cast a wide net over all of us. But the question is, "In what ways?" Some might seem obvious to you, while others might be more subtle. Some might be ever present, while others take advantage in a particular moment. I'd like you to consider: How has your fear of not belonging been exacerbated by media and society? How have you felt othered? Left out? Or so different that you needed to find some way to survive? Consider these prompts:

- One way I conformed growing up was _____.
- I felt pressure to _____ because I was _____.

- I needed to fit in because _____.
- The way that continues today is _____.

Exploring the origins of your belonging wound is no easy task. To identify the ways in which you've tried to fit in with others might bring up some emotion. Seeing the ways in which you traded authenticity to belong might activate something within you. Let that emotion motivate you. It doesn't need to stay that way. That's the beauty of this work; you get to choose a new path forward.

Coping with the Belonging Wound

To truly belong means that authenticity is in the driver's seat, not conformity. As the great Maya Angelou famously said, "You are only free when you realize you belong no place—you belong every place—no place at all." This is a profound moment of recognition. That when you belong to yourself, meaning you are at peace with yourself, you will simultaneously belong everywhere and nowhere. Everywhere is within you. Nowhere is outside of you. To be authentically yourself means that nothing can be taken from you, and that you relate to the threat of judgment, shaming, rejection, or disowning differently.

But few of us go directly from a belonging wound to sitting in acceptance of our authenticity. If only life were so easy. Rather we often take another, more harmful path first. We may walk the path of adaptation or rejection before we discover a way of belonging via being authentically ourselves.

THE PATH OF ADAPTATION

Most of us who are keenly aware of our differences start with adaptation. *Operate this way and you will belong.* Adaptation doesn't rock the boat, and it gives you what you crave in those early years: validation from the system around you. Rules, structure, and order have great value, and there's beauty to having a way of doing things in a family. On the healthy side of this, it's where belonging thrives. But when adaptation becomes a requirement, it intensifies. You get a false sense of belonging: *You're a part of the system, but only because you're changing who you really are.* This isn't belonging; this is fitting in.

When you try to fit in, you adapt to what the system is requiring of you for fear of the very real consequence: that if you don't, you won't belong. You might fear being treated differently, ignored, condescended to, degraded, or punished in some other way. Individuals, a community, or a system might judge you because of your differences. You understand that if you don't conform, you'll be out.

Many systems will ask you to adapt in order to fit in. A family may require you to meet their version of perfection in order to be one of them: for example, dressing a certain way, maintaining a particular image, or being a good little girl or boy. They might require you to always be agreeable, not to say another word when sharing an opinion, or never to talk about emotions or being upset. A cultural system may ask you to be more like the majority in order to be acknowledged, validated, respected, or even safe.

Adaptation, in this sense of trying to fit in is a path of survival, but it's not the destination. Ultimately, true belonging requires healing and evolution.

In what ways did you learn to survive through adaptation? You might think about this through the lens of your family, or you might think about this through the lens of the world at large. Can you see how adapting was of service to you before? Is it still of service to you or is it blocking something? There's no right or wrong answer here. Just open yourself up for reflection and observation.

THE PATH OF REJECTION

Rejection is when you consciously or unconsciously choose a path of opposition. This usually happens *after* you've participated in adaptation. Rejection is less an attempt at authenticity than it is an attempt at not being controlled, dominated, or chosen. It might appear and feel like you're taking a stand, but it's usually more of an angsty reactivity or rebellion than a grounded attempt at claiming your authenticity, ultimately pushing you to the outside even more.

Maybe you chose to dress or conduct yourself in a non-mainstream fashion. Maybe you acted out in ways that you knew were embarrassing to your family. Maybe you rejected a religion or the values that went along with it and took a path of being a nonbeliever in a family of devout believers. Either way, rejection generally leaves people feeling like they still are the outsider, the black sheep, and the one who doesn't belong.

Do you remember Carl, the navy brat from earlier in this chapter? When Carl first came to therapy, he wasn't coming in to talk about his controlling father. He came to see me because he was struggling with body image issues.

"I've been fat my entire life," he said to me in one of our sessions. "I've never felt attractive and I've never had anyone give me any type of positive attention. I want to believe that I can date, that someone will choose me, but it's really hard for me to trust that."

I could sense how painful this was for him. Carl described his entire family as super fit and expressed how difficult it was to be the fat one. I could of course understand why that was hard for him, but something felt off. I wanted to go back to understanding more about the militaristic mornings.

"Did you do the morning routine with your dad and your siblings throughout high school until you left for college?" I asked.

"No," he replied. "I stopped when I was about twelve."

"How'd that come about?" I asked.

"That's when I started getting fat," he said. "I couldn't do the drills because of all the extra weight I put on."

"I thought you said you had been fat your entire life," I responded.

"Well, yeah, I mean, I guess I just meant I was fat for most of my life. I was skinny before my dad moved home."

This detail was a big opening in our therapy together. Carl soon shared with me that he had put on the weight so that he physically *couldn't* do most of the things his father was drilling them to do. His verbal protests got him nowhere, but his weight gain finally put an end to it. Eventually Carl got so heavy that his father gave up and stopped paying attention to him altogether. Carl's unconscious attempt at making the military drills stop was successful, but it came at the cost of his feeling like he belonged in his family. He was no longer a part of the thing he didn't want to be part of, but he was also no longer a part of the family he *did* want to be a part of. It's interesting how whether you're in adaptation or rejection mode, you're still left feeling like you're on the outside, or at the very minimum, that you can't be authentically you.

Carl had found a path of rejection—one we both acknowledged was very creative, but that had still left him feeling even more ostracized. Carl was beginning to recognize that belonging wasn't about finding a way to fit in or reject his controlling father. Rather, it was about finding a way to choose himself.

The goal, as the late marriage and sex therapist Dr. David Schnarch suggests, is true differentiation, the ability to hold on to yourself while maintaining relationships with others. You stand up for yourself and what you believe in, but you do it in a calm way, not as a rebellion. Once you have this type of awareness, you no longer need the rebellion and rejection as a way of pushing back.

A path of rejection might be harder to spot than a path of adaptation, but I don't want you to miss how this path can still lead you to inauthenticity. When you rebel, your behaviors are still motivated by the pain of the avoidance, control, shame, and intolerance you once endured.

In what ways did you learn to survive through rejection? How has rejection served you? And does it still today? In what ways do you currently operate from a place of rejection, and might you get curious about what that's protecting you from or blocking you from?

THE PATH OF AUTHENTICITY

Living authentically means that your choices and actions align with your core beliefs, values, and true self. It means that you choose that path even when there are consequences from the world around you. We'll be discussing this further in chapter 11, "Making It Stick," but what I'd like to be very clear on here is that when there's a belonging wound at play, it's pretty hard to prioritize authenticity. Most people will find themselves either in adaptation or rejection for some time before they have a chance at truly honoring their authenticity.

Living authentically is uncomfortable if you haven't been living that way. It can shake your system in big ways because it means those who don't agree with you or those not living authentically themselves can't control or persuade you, can't shame or judge you into something, and their intolerance of you can't dictate your choices. Oof, that's some freedom.

When I met Neil, he wasn't living authentically. He was going along with the crowd, using drugs and sleeping around, even though the crowd wasn't pressuring him. He was betraying himself in order to get a taste of belonging. The moment it clicked that his behavior was connected to his belonging wound, Neil made a shift. He had felt abandoned by his family, and there was no way he was going to add to that by abandoning himself through decisions that were self-destructive. Neil wanted to fit in, but not at the expense of his health and his values. He wanted to belong, but he realized that he could never belong if he was being someone he wasn't.

Healing the Belonging Wound

In our work together, Neil's authenticity became something he would prioritize. When Neil was out partying but trying to call in a partner who wanted monogamy and a quiet, homey life, his system was calling bull. He had to begin to live the life he said he wanted, to truly embody it, before his values, his choices, and the results would align. If you say you want one thing but you choose to engage in things that directly conflict with that vision, it's hard for your system to trust what you say.

Although Neil rarely went back to West Virginia, when he was there for holidays, he let himself live out loud instead of in hiding. This came from a deeply grounded place. He wasn't attempting to embarrass his family or punish them in any way. He was simply living and allowing others to come face-to-face with what they would need to reconcile themselves. He was learning to belong to himself, to be who he was.

True belonging has no hint of arrogance or reactivity, and as Brené Brown says, it is not passive. "[True belonging] is a practice that requires us to be vulnerable, get uncomfortable, and learn how to be present with people without sacrificing who we are."

Vanessa, too, needed to exchange her false narrative of belonging through adaptation for a path of authenticity.

"No man is going to date a woman with a young child," she'd exclaim. And then follow it up with "And who's going to hire me after taking years off of work to raise my baby?" These narratives, among others, would keep her from dating, from applying for jobs, from moving, and from even sharing with people how she felt. She was unconsciously committed to not belonging. When I observed just that to her, she immediately became inquisitive.

"But why would I do that?" she asked.

"It serves something, doesn't it?" I responded.

She looked at me, a bit perplexed. I could see the wheels spinning—*Why would something serve me if it's not good for me?*—but then it clicked. "Does it serve my wounded parts? Like, it proves my origin wound right over and over again? And when I do that, I can just stay the same—I never have to create change."

Vanessa was getting it. To belong, truly, would ask her to change *everything*. By being herself. It's a task that is both hard work and also quite straightforward. She'd have to start getting clear on where *she* wanted to be, what was important to *her,* what inspired *her* and lit *her* up. And to stop letting fear and a lack of belonging lead her life. It meant finding peace within instead of seeking it outside of her. It meant showing up authentically, embracing herself, and dealing with the fears that would keep her from claiming things in her life that she wanted.

Life didn't look exactly the way that Vanessa wanted it to. But if she kept trying to prove a false story correct over and over again, life would never have a chance to look the way she wanted it to. Creating space for authenticity, for bravery and a belief in herself, set her on a path to finding her guiding light. Belonging was available to her at every moment, *in* any moment, as long as she let authenticity guide and lead her.

If you take a scan of your life right now, can you see where your choices and actions match with your core beliefs, values, and true self, and where they don't? Be gentle and honest with yourself here. If you were living authentically, what would be different?

- One way I betrayed myself for others growing up was _____.

- One way I still betray myself for others is _____.

The struggle to belong is never simple or easy. But the more Vanessa, Carl, Neil, Trish, and Bri explored their origin stories and did the work of noticing their belonging wound, witnessing it, grieving it, and pivoting from it, the more the grip their patterns had on them loosened. This isn't a tale of idealized stories. Vanessa would find herself stuck more times than she would like. Carl still struggled to believe that someone would find him attractive. It took years for Neil to find someone who wanted the same lifestyle as he did. Bri would catch herself shaming herself, and Trish still struggled to trust herself, especially when others would deny her cerebral palsy or question her. But what *did* happen is that Neil stopped pretending and did a much better job at saying no to things that were a no. Carl changed his relationship to his self-image and saw a path forward where belonging didn't require being controlled. Vanessa began making changes in her life that allowed her to be a part of things bigger than herself. Bri increasingly noticed her inner critic and was able to offer herself compassion and grace. Trish strengthened her relationship with self-trust. This work is a forever commitment. It must happen over and over again. That became the work, and so their healing began.

Origin Healing Practice

Let's take the work a bit further. If a belonging wound resonated with you, let's work through the Origin Healing Practice together.

Get comfortable. You might lie down or sit on a chair. Your eyes can be open or closed. Make sure your setting feels safe and private. As a reminder, if you're moving through trauma, it's vital you take good care. Having someone who can guide you, support you, and help create a safe space for you while you do this work is necessary.

NAMING Can you bring into focus the first time you questioned whether you belonged? Just notice the first time you were or felt like an outsider. Do you remember the day? Do you remember where you were? Do you remember who made you question it? See how many details you can name.

WITNESSING Now become more focused on yourself. Try zooming in on the younger version of yourself as you experience your belonging wound for the first time. And as if you were watching yourself on a video, I want you to notice the feelings you experienced in that moment. Notice the expression on your face, notice any change in body language. And begin to let yourself feel for that little child, the younger you.

GRIEVING You might begin to feel emotion start to surface. Can you let it come? You might be attuned to what it must have been like for you all those years earlier. Your heart might break for your younger self who had to endure the belonging wound. Go ahead and feel for that child. Maybe you notice the emotion around the ways you adapted to fit in, or the rebellious stand you took and what that felt like back then. Just notice what you want to offer your younger self in this moment. Do you want to hug her? Do you want to tell him that you're so sorry he ever had to go through that? Do you want to pick them up and tell them it's going to be okay? What are you feeling compelled to do? And just notice that.

Be here for as long or as little feels comfortable to you. If your eyes are closed, take some time before you enter back into the room. Keep your eyes closed and bring some movement back into your fingertips, into your toes. Maybe you stretch your neck. Maybe you put your hands on your heart or your belly. Maybe you bring awareness back into your breath. Think about what you'll see when you open your eyes. Can you remember where you are? And ever so slowly, flutter your eyes open. Take your time here.

Remember, you can do this as many times as you need, as you want. You may do this every day for a week. Or you might do it once and come back next year or in five years. I am so proud of you.

PIVOTING As we come to an end, I'd love for you to take a moment to acknowledge how your belonging wound shows up today. In what ways? In what relationships? Can you finish this sentence? *If I allowed myself to live authentically, if I wasn't afraid to just be, what would be different is* _____. For this week I'd like you to see if you can just notice when there would be an opportunity to replace an old way with a new way. Just notice. There's nothing more you need to do now.

As always, hand on heart . . . you're doing it. Take a moment to acknowledge yourself for all that you are allowing yourself to see and feel.

5

I WANT TO BE PRIORITIZED

Children don't directly ask their parents to prioritize them. They don't use those exact words. Instead, they ask their parents to play with them, go outside with them, or read to them. These are their bids for connection and prioritization. If they're using their words, they might say something like "No work, Mama," or "Bad TV" or "No more phone." The things that distract parents from children are at best stressors to that child, and at worst threaten children's beliefs about themselves and their value in this world. Later in life, the children of chronically distracted parents may consciously believe they are seeking out relationships in which they are a priority. In reality, however, these still-wounded adults wind up unconsciously seeking out dynamics that tend to repeat and support what they learned from their families decades earlier: they don't matter.

If you didn't feel prioritized in your family system, then you might have a prioritization wound. A prioritized child is a child whose needs are seen, understood, and honored. It doesn't mean that you're given everything you want or that you're the focus in every moment. Parents are allowed to have boundaries and say no, and they're allowed to have a life of their own that they, too, honor and prioritize. But what it does mean is that your parents tune into you. They listen, they care, they're curious, they notice, and they prioritize what's happening in your inner and outer world. You might not like the decisions they make for you at times, but you don't question whether you matter or are important to them.

When prioritization is in question, it's because you're given messages that you begin to decipher and then incorporate into your belief system. Sometimes those messages are explicit, like parents repeatedly telling you to leave them alone or saying things like "It's Sunday! Don't bother your father while he watches his football." Other times the messages are implicit, like a parent ignoring you while you're speaking or parents who are constantly in conflict making little room for you to ask for help on your homework or to watch a movie together. A prioritization wound leaves you questioning your importance and value to the people to whom you so desperately want to matter.

Origins of the Prioritization Wound

When a couple comes to see me, I'm often playing detective. The couple will describe their conflict in those first sessions and often want to share all the details. They'll talk about the fights they have and try to prove their point to me. They're testing to see whose side I might lean toward or gauge how bad I think it is. "Can our relationship be saved? Have you seen any other couple with this?" they might ask.

Of course there's value in hearing some of the details, but that initial airing of the story is rarely complete. What they think they're showing up to therapy for is just the tip of the iceberg. To pinpoint what's really being activated in the relationship usually requires a deeper dive, one that asks us to investigate their families and uncover their origin wounds.

When Isabel and Josefina first came to me, they, like most couples beginning their therapy, were focused on proving their point and try-ing to find a quick solution. I met both of them two years after they'd moved to New York City together from Spain. They'd both been ac-cepted into a graduate program they were excited to attend. When former friends become lovers, this can often lead to beautiful rela-tionships, but Isabel and Josefina had hit a rough patch in theirs and were struggling with recurring conflict that never seemed to get re-solved.

They came in for their first session together and I could immedi-ately feel their nerves.

"Does it matter where we sit?" Isabel asked.

I pointed to the sofa and let them choose their spots. Isabel sat closest to me. And although Josefina wasn't too far away, it was Isabel who was directly in front. I noted their positions.

"Thanks for coming in. I'd love to hear from both of you why you're here today."

Not surprisingly, Isabel started. "We've been fighting a lot lately. Really this whole last year. And we can't fix anything. It feels like we're just getting further and further away from each other, and it scares me. Jo has been talking about breaking up and I don't want that, but I also don't know what to do."

"Can you tell me what you fight about?"

"Well, it's me who is mostly complaining about Jo. When we first moved here from Spain, it felt so exciting for us to be doing this ad-venture together. Neither one of us had ever lived anywhere else, so it felt like we were setting off on some joint voyage. Our first year here was good. We lived together and started making friends in our pro-gram and pretty much were inseparable, but now she's been doing more things on her own, which is fine, but it doesn't seem like she even wants me around. She stays out late, we barely spend time to-gether, and she responds less frequently to my texts."

Isabel paused for a moment. I was looking at her while she was speaking, but I always check in on the other partner to see if I can notice any facial or body expressions that might show up as they listen to their partner share their perspective. Jo was distant and closed off. She seemed annoyed to even be there. She would roll her eyes from time to time and very subtly shake her head in irritation as she listened to Isabel. I knew it was only a matter of time before she released a rant that would give us some more information.

"Josefina, do you prefer if I call you Jo?" I asked.

"You can call me whatever you want. Jo is for the people who know me well, but I imagine you're going to know me really well pretty soon here, so you might as well just start calling me that now."

She had some attitude, for sure, but there was an invitation there letting me know that she was open to me getting to know her well.

When I asked Jo what had changed for her, she was able to articulate it clearly. She agreed that Isabel had been her best friend and that things were great their first year in New York City. But Jo quickly started to feel smothered by Isabel. Jo had started to make her own friends and would go out without Isabel. Isabel continued to want to do everything together. Jo felt Isabel was trying to keep her life small, and when she felt controlled by Isabel, she admitted that things got heated. They would argue and find themselves never coming to a resolution. Jo made it very clear that having a life outside of her relationship was a nonnegotiable. She needed her space for her health. She had been in codependent relationships before and she wasn't going to engage in anything similar to that ever again. Jo loved Isabel, but she felt herself getting more disconnected and shutting down.

This wasn't the first time that Isabel was hearing Jo express this. Even though it made her sad, a part of her seemed to understand.

I saw two women in front of me who had taken on quite the adventure with each other. They had bravely decided to go on an exciting journey to a country neither of them had ever been to before in pursuit of a similar dream. When you engage in big transitions, you inevitably have certain unstated expectations and fantasies about how the whole experience might go. Dr. Robert Glover, author of *No More Mr. Nice Guy!*, calls these unstated assumptions *covert expectations,* the unspoken agreements we *think* we have in the relationship and with our partner. It seemed to me as if Isabel and Jo were struggling with a vision collision and an expectation crisis.

Isabel was struggling to feel like a priority in Jo's life. She was questioning whether she even mattered to Jo. Isabel was devastated by this thought, given they had been each other's person for so long. It *is* really gut-wrenching when the person you love doesn't want to spend the time with you that you want to spend with them. Isabel was doing everything in her power to get Jo to make her a priority, from begging and pleading to pretending it didn't matter to her, from ultimatums to full-on tantrums. In our sessions, Isabel would get angry and lash out at Jo any time Jo would assert her desire for independence and autonomy.

Isabel's reactivity in our session was a good indicator that there was more to uncover. If you remember from chapter 2, reactivity is like a neon sign with an arrow pointing toward your fears, insecurities, and doubts. It lets us know that something important predates this specific moment and that we ought to learn about it. We began to identify the wound that was being activated.

In our second session, I asked Isabel whether she had felt like a priority in her family.

"Oh yes, of course, my family loves me so much."

I wasn't convinced. Of course she could have developed this wound later in life, but I got a sense that someone had deprioritized her when she was growing up. That neon sign was blinking. Not feeling like a priority with Jo was not the first time that Isabel had felt that emotion.

"Can you tell me about your mom? I'd love to know how you would describe her as an individual, but also how she was as a mother to you."

"She was a good mother. She stayed home with me and my siblings, and I always had fun with her. She was playful and a really good caretaker. Everyone loved my mom; she was the life of the party. But she became very sad at one point."

"What happened?" I asked.

"When I was seven, my mom's sister died of suicide. I didn't know what had actually happened at the time, I just knew that she had died, but everything changed after that. My mom fell into a depression and never came out of it, still to this day. It was so sad to see her like that. It was like the life really got sucked out of her. She had been such a vibrant woman, and after this, she didn't do anything. She would barely leave her bed and her room. My father had to take on a lot. He was very loving with her and we took care of her together."

Jo was looking at Isabel. She had heard this story before, but this time she was actually taking it in.

Isabel's mother's depression became a priority in her family. It was all-consuming. Of course her mother didn't want this—it just happened. They knew she was sad, but no action was taken. Her father, who was the salt of the earth, did what he could. He worked two jobs, cooked and cleaned, and cared for his wife as best he could. But he was ill equipped to handle all this, to say the least.

I was struck by how significant this story was in understanding the pain that Isabel was reliving as a twenty-nine-year-old woman in New York City. During Isabel's first seven years she'd experienced joy, connection, love, and some serious prioritization as the baby of the family. She was at the center of the family system, with hands-on older siblings and two parents who really loved her. Of course, she said she was a priority in her family when I asked her. But she was speaking only of the first few years in her life.

After her aunt's death, everything changed. Not only was she not the focus, but she also had to be deprioritized. As Isabel told me, "My father didn't know how to ask for help from anyone other than me. I think he was ashamed and wanted to protect my mom, so he didn't want anyone to see her that way."

Jo and I got it. There was nothing malicious here. This was a case of a devastating event taking place that affected the entire family so significantly that Isabel, a seven-year-old girl, could no longer be a priority in her parent's lives—even if they wished otherwise.

This event laid the foundation for Isabel's prioritization wound. Her mother's mental health became the priority in her father's life as well as in her own. She helped her father cook, clean, and care for her mom. It was common to hear him say, "Can you go try to cheer your mother up? I think she would really like you to spend time with her." And this was true, of course—it was helpful for her mom—but what was also true was that as Isabel took on the tasks of cooking, cleaning, and cheering up her mom, there wasn't space for her to be a little girl with very real developmental, physical, emotional, and experiential needs to be met.

Isabel had never thought about her life and her family this way. What struck her even more was recognizing that the drastic change she was feeling in the relationship with Jo felt quite similar to what she had experienced with her family. She had been in a situation where she was the priority, and then things changed dramatically, and her needs were no longer taken into account.

I could see Jo softening a bit. She uncrossed her arms and dropped her shoulders. This information didn't change the fact that she didn't want to be controlled, but she was seeing Isabel in a new light, one that added layers of context and clarity.

Isabel had never realized that she didn't feel like a priority in her family. That version of the story felt unfair because of the beautiful family life she had once had. She understood that her parents had few resources and were truly doing the best they could. She preferred connecting to the life she had before things had changed. The family stories she liked to recount to Jo were the version of her mother and family that she wanted to remember and share with others. Speaking of how life was after her mother's depression was more painful, so she avoided talking about it, connecting to it, and understanding its lasting effects until our therapy together.

Identifying her prioritization wound wasn't something Isabel was necessarily excited about, especially as it meant reshaping her narrative about her past into a less-than-happy one. But this step was necessary in order to figure out how this unhealed origin wound was helping drive her and Jo apart.

I've met countless individuals with a prioritization wound. Their stories reveal preoccupied and distracted parents who consistently prioritized themselves over their children. And their stories reveal caretakers who were struggling with their own unhealed origin wounds that prevented them from showing up fully and prioritizing their children.

Even though I focus on familial origin stories below, I want to remind you that your prioritization wound might have shown up later in life, and it may have initiated through relationships outside of your family of origin. You might realize that the first time you felt deprioritized in a wounding way was with a former partner or in a meaningful friendship instead of with a family member. Keep your mind open as we explore this together.

A PREOCCUPIED AND DISTRACTED FAMILY OF ORIGIN

Preoccupation and distraction are cut from the same cloth. When your parents or other members of your extended family are engrossed in something else—when they are distracted or preoccupied—they are rarely giving their full attention to a child. The distraction could be the result of an ongoing issue—a parent's relationship to their work, for example—or of all-consuming challenges—alcohol or drug abuse, gambling, mental or physical health issues. Or it could be something that consumes them for specific periods, like having marital problems over a period of a couple of years or being easily overwhelmed by emotions.

Andrei's prioritization wound developed because he was the child of a single mother who worked two jobs just to get by. Andrei was always so kind and loving when he described his mother. I could tell how much he loved and respected her, but when he was little, all he wanted was time with her that he couldn't have. She worked double shifts six days a week to provide for them, and he got to see her only on Sundays, when they would go to church and have lunch together before her evening shift started.

Andrei was immensely grateful to his mother for her sacrifices on his behalf, and indeed at times would rationalize that working double shifts *was* her way of prioritizing him. But this never changed the fact that what he craved the most was time with her. The wound was there, even though she was doing everything in her power to set him up for a better future.

Of course origin wounding can show up even when a person or family is well intentioned. We'd like to think that it has to come from maliciousness or negligence, when the reality is it can show up in countless other ways, where no bad intentions are present.

This was true for Khaite's mom, who also was preoccupied with challenges in her own life. Khaite's parents never got married; her father had found someone who was a better match for him, or so he said, when Khaite was only four years old. Her mother was devastated by this rejection, and subsequently became obsessed with dating and finding love with a new partner. There were times when it seemed like she was going on dates every other night.

"She would come home from these dates and tell me everything about them. I don't think she realized that she would never ask me questions about myself when she was dating. She got so lost in it all," Khaite recalled. She loved her mother very much, but this was still painful for her. She never wanted to make her mom feel bad, but she also wasn't interested in having "girl talk" with her parent. She wanted her mom to show consistent interest in *her* life; she wanted to feel important to her mom, not to be dropped to the bottom of the priority list as these men came in and out of their lives. Khaite wanted so badly to be a priority, but her mother's preoccupation with her own love life was blocking that.

A chronically distracted and preoccupied family has lasting effects. It's painful to grow up questioning whether you're a priority, whether you matter more than those other things that are distracting the adults from paying attention to you. And that experience can come forward with you into your adult relationships, in ways that are both obvious and subtle.

PARENTS' UNRESOLVED WOUNDS

During the period when you were growing up, the adults in your life likely experienced wounds of their own. In fact, they might still have wounds that are unacknowledged and unresolved to this day. These wounds can easily get passed on to you. Maybe they prioritized themselves because they themselves were not prioritized as children. Maybe they put their own needs, wants, and desires first, above yours, because they were overlooked when they were growing up. There are endless ways a parent's unresolved wounds can be passed on. This perspective offers important context, but it doesn't change the fact that you didn't feel prioritized. It is never the child's responsibility to manage and navigate the unhealed wounds of their parents, but unfortunately, this happens far too often.

Sarah had shared with me that when she was a child, she was obsessed with photography. She wanted to learn everything there was to know about it. She had begged and pleaded for a camera for her eleventh birthday and had received the best of the best. But two years after she'd received that exciting gift, her parents sat her down to tell her that she could no longer pursue her interest in photography. "They said it was 'beneath me' and I needed to focus on skills that would get me into 'the right' college," she said.

Sarah's parents were wealthy. She grew up on the Upper East Side of Manhattan, and her parents outlined a specific plan for her both educationally and professionally. They told her that there was no money in photography—after all, it was just a hobby—and she needed to start taking her future seriously. This was devastating for her. Even speaking about it decades later, she shook her head, immense heartache obvious on her face.

Her parents had plenty of resources to help Sarah with her dream. They simply refused to accept it because of the humiliation they felt they'd suffer in their circles if she didn't follow a more prescribed career path. "They wanted me to be a doctor," she said. "I remember a very specific moment before we attended some holiday party with all their friends when they told me not to mention my dreams of photography to anyone. My mom literally said, 'Please don't embarrass us tonight.' They were reacting to what others would think of them as parents and cared more about that than about what made me light up in this world." This revealed *their* anxieties and fears—really, *their* belonging wounds—and though they didn't see it this way, their actions prioritized their needs above Sarah's.

It was heartbreaking to hear this story. Sarah had gone on to become a very successful doctor. She hated her profession, but what she hated even more was how miserable she was. She came to see me because her boyfriend had just broken up with her for the fourth time. They kept getting back together because the love was there, but they struggled to resolve what she called a deal breaker: he wanted kids and she was a maybe.

As we dug in, I learned that Sarah actually *did* want kids. But she was unconsciously testing her ex to see whether he would be willing to put her wishes first, something her parents never did. There was a lot to unpack, but this realization opened up so much for Sarah. Her prioritization wound—the feeling that she was never number one in the eyes of those she loved—was still having a profound impact on her in the present day.

There might be some unresolved wounds that exist in your family system that contributed to your prioritization wound. And while this is never about making excuses, can you get curious about whether family members' unhealed pain kept them from prioritizing you?

Origin wound identification isn't meant to offer an excuse. It doesn't make reactivity okay; it just makes it make sense. Origin wound identification also isn't the end. It's a jumping-off point, the catalyst that begins to move you toward healing.

Coping with the Prioritization Wound

Many children work tirelessly at being prioritized, doing everything they can to figure out who they need to be or what they need to do in order to be prioritized by their caretakers. But when their efforts fail, eventually they throw in the towel and accept their de-prioritized status. My heart breaks at the thought that a child might need to concede to this. When this happens in childhood, that manner of coping may extend into adulthood.

THE PATH OF REPETITION

As we've seen previously, one way we often cope with our wounds is to unintentionally repeat them in our adult relationships. This was true for both Andrei and Khaite.

In the psychology world we have a theory about something called the intergenerational transmission of psychopathology. (I know, it's a mouthful, but I promise I'm keeping the jargon to a minimum.) This is the genetic and nongenetic transfer of behaviors, characteristics, and traits from generation to generation. Simpler version: A lot is transferred to us from the generations before us. And not surprisingly, we often repeat what it is we observed or experienced growing up.

Have you ever heard someone say some version of "you're just like your mother or father" either about you or about someone you know? In fact, maybe you've said those words out loud yourself. The path of repetition is a straightforward and obvious one. You repeat the behaviors, characteristics, and traits of those who came before you. This can happen without your being aware of it, like growing up with an angry and reactive parent just to find yourself angry and reactive decades later. And sometimes this happens despite your best efforts, like growing up in an abusive home and swearing to yourself that you will never abuse your own child, only to find yourself repeating the cycle. Both Andrei and Khaite found themselves taking a path of repetition when it came to their prioritization wound in their adult relationships—one unconsciously, the other more aware of what was happening but repeating the cycle nonetheless.

Andrei, whose mother sacrificed everything for him yet whose double shifts left him with a prioritization wound, showed up to therapy saying that his wife was making him go because she was fed up with his playing video games after work. He maintained that this was his way of decompressing. Through our work together, Andrei realized that video games were his second shift. He had revealed to me that he would play upward of six hours a night. Instead of choosing partners who were preoccupied, *he* was the preoccupied one, ultimately putting his wife in his childhood position and repeating his prioritization wound by distracting himself. By doing this, he not only maintained his wound but left his wife feeling de-prioritized as well. Sometimes when we believe that we can't be prioritized, we create an environment that keeps us in that position.

While Andrei was at first oblivious to the ways he was repeating his prioritization wound, Khaite immediately recognized her patterns. She owned right away that she was distracted in her relationship and confessed to spending hours at night scrolling on Instagram. This was cutting into her time with her partner and affecting their intimacy.

"I know, I know. I'm doing the same thing my mom did to me," Khaite said matter-of-factly. She saw it, but she also continued to engage in the behavior. Her awareness was not enough for her to change what she knew, but it was enough to engage us in a dialogue about what was playing out.

Khaite had never shared with her mother how much she had felt de-prioritized. And because of that, Khaite never heard her mother acknowledge the distractions and take accountability—something Khaite needed to hear. Instead, Khaite had unconsciously repeated the same pattern, putting her former partner in the same position Khaite had been in with her mom. If her partner could have the same experiences Khaite had had all those years ago, Khaite believed she would feel seen, understood, and validated. Once we identified this, she saw how harmful it was to their dynamic. She didn't actually *want* her partner to feel de-prioritized; she wanted to feel heard and understood. She realized that there was a better way of going about making that happen.

Fortunately, Khaite did have a receptive mother. In our work together, Khaite summoned up the courage to bring this to her mom. Her mom was able to validate her experience, take ownership, and wholeheartedly apologize for being so distracted. That former little girl had been witnessed; this was incredibly healing for Khaite. But Khaite's additional healing required her, too, to take ownership, to apologize to her partner for passing on the pain, and to make significant shifts toward being present and prioritizing her partner and the relationship.

The path of repetition may seem obvious, but it's easy to miss. You may have proclaimed things years ago about how you'd never do this or that, but I've met so many folks who don't even realize that they are behaving in the same ways they swore they never would. This path is easily recognizable, but sometimes it hides in plain sight. If you really open your eyes wide, what might you see?

THE PATH OF OPPOSITION

The more subtle transmission of behaviors from generation to generation at first looks like the exact opposite of repetition. It involves doing the exact opposite of what we observed and experienced. If you really hated or disliked something while you were growing up, it's no wonder you'd want to take a different path. When you witness pain, devastation, or behaviors you despise, you sensibly might want to do a one-eighty as a way to protect yourself or set yourself up for what you see as success. Maybe you saw alcohol ruin your mother's life and you've committed to never touching the stuff. Maybe you grew up in a family where conflict was ever present, and now you avoid conflict at all costs. Or maybe your parents overspent and went into debt, so now you're frugal with your own spending. There are plenty of ways we take a path of opposition to those who came before us. And from the outside looking in, it might appear to be a healthier path to take. Who's going to argue with a person choosing not to drink or

THE ORIGINS OF YOU

someone who avoids conflict or a person who saves more than he spends? These all come across as sound decisions. But if they're a path of opposition due to an unhealed wound, fear is running the show and making the decisions for you. And a path of opposition causes many issues, as you can see in Isabel and Jo's story.

Isabel's countless demands on Jo were in many ways a path of opposition to being de-prioritized. She didn't want to be treated as an adult the way she had been as a child. She was going to try to demand prioritization from others, especially Jo. *The way to be prioritized is to make others prioritize me.* Isabel pressured Jo to choose her over all else. But this tactic only worked against her. The more Isabel pushed, the more Jo disconnected. Once Isabel identified and noticed her prioritization wound and the path of opposition she was on, she was able to see her behavior differently.

Isabel's prioritization wound was also getting activated by what she was experiencing as Jo's selfishness. Let me just state right now that a desire for autonomy is not selfish. A desire to have a life separate from your partner is not the problem. In fact, we know couples in satisfying relationships balance autonomy and a sense of togetherness by supporting each other's individual dreams while also creating shared meaning as a couple. Jo's desire to spend time with her own friends without Isabel wasn't innately bad or wrong. Her desire to check out events without having Isabel by her side didn't have to mean that she wasn't prioritizing Isabel.

The problem was that issues were left unaddressed for so long that Jo *was* operating from a selfish place. Isabel, in return, would lash out, call Jo names, and leave messages demanding Jo return home by a certain time or not bother coming home. Jo had gotten so fed up with Isabel's increasingly angry demands for attention and prioritization that she did lack consideration and concern for Isabel. Jo had begun prioritizing her own fun even when she knew that Isabel was at home crying herself to sleep. That might sound harsh, but this wasn't because Jo was a terrible person; this was because Jo and Isabel had let things build up in their relationship without properly communicating. Over time each grew resentful of the other, and they slipped into a dynamic that kept re-creating a pattern of de-prioritization for Isabel even as Isabel tried to counter the pattern from her childhood and seize control.

When we feel threatened, we generally do whatever we can to make sure we don't reexperience the same thing that initiated the pain. *If our relationship changes, then I can't be the priority.* This thought was one that had been coming to a head in the relationship with Jo. Isabel didn't mean to be controlling, but she *was* being controlling. Trying to stop Jo from hanging with her friends or spending any time away was Isabel's attempt at creating safety for herself, but it was backfiring badly.

What Isabel didn't realize was that she needed to do her own origin healing work or the wound would never heal. She couldn't rely on Jo to treat it for her. If Jo just went along with what Isabel was asking for, she might help Jo temporarily soothe her prioritization wound, but Isabel's wound would just keep reopening, and Jo would likely grow even more resentful. Jo would be living life in order to please and relieve her partner at the expense of her own reasonable desire for autonomy and interdependence. This approach doesn't work, and we have the research to show it. Now more than ever, the fundamental purpose of marriage, of relationships, is for partners to help each other meet their needs for autonomy and personal growth.

You may have worked hard at becoming a priority in your family. Maybe your efforts succeeded at times when you traded your authenticity, or maybe they fell flat and you gave up. How you learned to cope back then may be the same ways you cope now. Maybe you've repeated the pattern by de-prioritizing others in your life, or maybe you've been committed to a path of opposition, one where you do everything in your power to make sure you don't experience what you once did. But what you might be recognizing is that none of this actually leaves you feeling prioritized. It doesn't actually heal the wound. It just rubs salt in it.

Healing the Prioritization Wound

You may have already worked through the Origin Healing Practice for yourself in one of the previous chapters, but I want you to get to experience the power of reading how someone else—in this case, Isabel—worked through her practice with me in session. Remember, to be witness to someone else's process is an honor. As you read, notice what comes up for you. How do you feel about Isabel and the way she works through this practice? Does it teach you something? Do you notice yourself judging something? What do you take away from being so intimate with someone else's healing process?

Once Isabel understood her need to heal her prioritization wound, the sessions that followed were profound. Isabel was able to close her eyes, bring her seven-year-old self into focus in her imagination, and witness her. Setting all distractions aside, Isabel was able to fully honor her younger self as she was. It's an incredible act of reclamation after a long time spent minimizing, rationalizing, or invalidating her experience. Lives quite literally change when witnessing happens.

On this day, Jo and I were witness to Isabel as she spoke out loud what it was like to be an observer of her own self over two decades earlier. I often describe this exercise to my clients as pulling up a chair to your little you, however old she might be, and getting close enough to see the details but far enough away to avoid crossing a physical boundary. Can you envision it? The house? The top of the stairs you used to perch on? Your bedroom? Of course, it's not always a single disturbing event like what Isabel experienced. If you were de-prioritized chronically—perhaps with a parent who was always working or was getting drunk every night—then you can bring one or multiple visuals forward for you to witness, observe, and tune into.

"Isabel, is it okay if I guide you here a bit?" I asked.

"Sure," she answered hesitantly.

All three of us took breaths together with our eyes closed in order to ground ourselves in the room.

"Can you bring little Isabel into focus and tell me about her? What's she wearing right now? What does she look like?"

"She has long brown hair that's in two braids. Gosh, I loved to wear braids. And she's wearing a T-shirt and purple shorts and sneakers."

"Can you see her face? What do you notice?"

"She's smiling, but I can tell that she's actually quite sad behind the smile."

"Does she see you sitting next to her yet? Can you let her know that you're with her?"

"Sure." Isabel paused for a moment. "Hi," she said to her younger self.

Isabel began to cry. She no longer needed any guidance from me. She continued: "Hi, sweet girl. I'm so sorry that life changed for you so significantly in what felt like a blink of an eye. Your life was special, and I'm so sorry that you lost so many of your favorite people so quickly. I know they were still there, but they weren't. I'm so sorry you couldn't be prioritized. I'm so sorry that depression filled the home and that you and Dad started to become responsible for things that you shouldn't have had to take on. I'm so sorry. You've been working so hard to get people to prioritize you, but the way you're going about it isn't giving you what you need. I'm so sorry I haven't been able to see that sooner. I'm sorry I haven't been able to guide you, us, better. I will."

Isabel took a breath. My eyes were still closed, but I cracked them to take a peek to see what was happening with both Jo and Isabel.

Jo had taken Isabel's hand and I could see the remainder of tears on her face. She had moved closer to Isabel, and Isabel's head was resting on Jo's shoulder. When I looked at Isabel, I saw a woman who was fully transported. She was deeply present to her seven-year-old self. It was in this moment that Isabel stepped into prioritizing herself. As she safely named and witnessed the wound and how she adapted to it, she disconnected from it and began to prioritize herself. And because Jo and I were also present, she had the experience of having others witness both adult her and little her. This was something that Isabel did many times in session, but also an intentional practice she often did by herself at home.

Isabel was also learning to feel her grief, which meant that she was learning to feel love as well. Grief and love are conjoined, as author Jandy Nelson says. We don't experience one without the other. To continue resisting grief would mean to resist self-love. As Isabel created intentional space to grieve, she was simultaneously creating space to love herself. Note, this isn't about *forcing* grief. You are allowed to choose not to go there. In fact, we do that often as a healthy way to cope. But there will come a time when you can't ignore the feelings. Grief will continue to knock on your door in obvious and subtle ways. Not because it wants to torture you, but because it wants to be relieved.

For Isabel, this work wasn't about getting over something, but rather about relating to it differently. She couldn't change what had had happened, but she could change the hold it had on her, something that her mom had never quite figured out. When we sit with our grief and learn how to spend time with it, the hurt and harm we feel from the past doesn't need to resurface every time something familiar shows up. Isabel had put the responsibility on Jo to comfort her and to make her a priority, in an unconscious attempt to avoid having to feel the loneliness of being in a new city without lots of friends and the anticipatory sadness of not feeling important enough to her partner. This was a subtle reenactment of what Isabel had experienced as a little girl when she'd been asked to adjust and be the comfort for her mom because the adults were preoccupied with their own wounds. This was all eye-opening, but it happened only because Isabel was willing to go *there*.

The couple needed to see that had Jo just gone along with Isabel's requests for prioritization, she actually wouldn't have been doing much good for Isabel. Of course, the way Jo was handling things also wasn't doing much good, but that was for us to work out in the pivot.

The pivot, as you know, is where the rubber meets the road. This is where you move your knowing into doing. It's the opportunity to choose a different way of responding even when the things around you are familiar. The pivot happens in the space between being activated (or triggered) and your reaction. There's a moment in between when you have an opportunity to change your normal pattern of behavior. Instead of being led by your unconscious programming, where your conditioning takes over, you're led by your awareness. In the pivot you take a moment, or many, to recall what you've already identified as a pattern and lead yourself forward on a path of responsiveness instead of one of reactivity. It is absolutely easier said than done, and that becomes your life's practice.

Isabel needed to notice when her prioritization wound was getting activated and to pause to name it, witness it, and grieve it so that she would have more clarity on what needed to happen next. For a pivot to take place, she needed to be clear with herself and clear in her expression with her partner. Instead of criticizing Jo, Isabel would need to bring her emotional need into the open. You'll learn more about this in chapter 8, "Conflict," but for now it's enough for you to recognize that when the focus changes from criticism and complaints to an airing of emotional needs, a couple has a much better shot at pivoting together and ending up at a different outcome.

When I mentioned that they would need to pivot together, Jo

asked, "So what do we do? What do we do when I want to go spend time with friends on my own? I don't want Isabel to feel de-prioritized. I'm not trying to hurt her, but I do want to be able to have some space for myself and for her to have that, too."

Jo was doing it. She just didn't realize it. The very fact that she named that she didn't want Isabel to feel de-prioritized was such a beautiful first step. She was acknowledging with Isabel that she was aware of the wound and didn't want to intentionally activate it with her. She was mindful that doing things that historically made Isabel feel de-prioritized still felt a little troublesome.

This would be our continued work together. From Jo communicating her individual plans but reminding Isabel that she was indeed a priority, to Isabel working on depersonalizing the fact that Jo wanted to do things without her from time to time. Their growth was beautiful to witness.

Isabel's pivot work also required her to find ways to self-soothe when her wound was activated by Jo's independence. I suggested she replace her old behaviors with new ones. Instead of angrily texting Jo, she might read a book, call a friend, or go for a walk. By self-soothing and substituting new behaviors for old, she'd find ways to calm herself without resorting to demands on Jo.

We worked week in and week out on their identifying, witnessing, and grieving when something felt familiar, and they both worked hard at noticing the space for the pivot and communicating what was happening in their inner worlds. A great way to do this is by narrating your inner thoughts. When Isabel would find the pivot, she might say to Jo, "I know that it's important for you to go see your friends, but the story I'm telling myself is that I'm not a priority to you." This was a page out of Narrative Therapy work, which was largely developed by Michael White and David Epston in the seventies and eighties. This work focuses the individual on developing stories about themselves and their identities that are helpful to them, instead of

authoring ones that aren't. In Isabel and Jo's case, Isabel's articula-
tion of the negative story she was telling herself, that she wasn't a
priority, gave Jo space to disrupt that story. Jo might respond by saying, "Thanks for sharing that with me. That story isn't true. You are
absolutely a priority to me. I love you and I can't wait to spend time
with you tomorrow. I'll have my phone on me and I'll check in
throughout the night." This might sound idealized to you. You might
even be rolling your eyes, thinking, *Who speaks that way?!* And I get
it, but Jo and Isabel were able to utilize their pivot this way because
they worked really hard to get there. It wasn't perfect, but it was progress. Don't forget that they started where you might be.

Of course we all entertain in our minds endless stories about what
another person is feeling, thinking, or perceiving. A valuable prompt
originally from Narrative Therapy but made famous by Brené Brown
in her book *Rising Strong* is "The story I'm telling myself is . . ." Perhaps you can use this prompt to get clear with yourself but also to
share your story and check it, the way Isabel did above, with the other
person so it opens up dialogue instead of supporting silent rumina-
tion and uncertainty. Give it a shot and see what it does.

There are likely many differences between your healing practice
and Isabel's, but one significant one that might stand out is that you
may not be working through any of this with a partner. You might
not have a Jo by your side doing some of the witnessing with you. But
if you do have a partner or close family member or friend you'd like
to invite into this intimate space with you, something special and
healing might happen.

This is not required, of course, but it may be very helpful, especially if an origin wound has led to relational wounding in the present
day. Origin relational wounding, a wound that comes from a relationship, convinces us that we need another human being to disprove the
message that we were given in our childhoods. You might be like so
many others who convince themselves that the proof of their

importance or value lies in the hands of someone else—that it lives outside them, not within them. *I'm a priority when someone shows me that I'm a priority. I'm worthy once someone tells me I am. I belong once I fit in with the group.* It makes sense why we'd think that way. And here's the catch: To some degree, you *do* need relationships to assist in that healing. I'm a big believer that if relationships wound, then relationships must assist in the healing. But this work is both relational and individual. Even though you might not start off by seeking a deep inner knowing and peace around your value, your worthiness, or your belonging all on your own, it's a direction you need to consider.

Origin Healing Practice

Let's do a little work if you're up for it. I will always remind you to take good care of yourself as you work through your exploration. Pause if necessary. Your job is not to push through and force.

> NAMING Remember that noticing or identifying a prioritization wound does not require you to betray or discount the love you *did* receive from a family member.
>
> Can you bring into focus the first time you questioned whether you were a priority in your family? It might be with someone specific or it might be with the whole family system. Do you remember who made you question it? Do you remember where you were that first time? What you were doing? Or what you wanted that other person to do or say? Do you remember what or who was more important than prioritizing you? See how many details you can notice.

WITNESSING Try zooming in on the younger version of yourself that you're witnessing feeling de-prioritized for the first time or the subsequent times. Pull up that chair close enough to see the details on your face, your expression, and your body language. And begin to let yourself feel for that little child, younger you.

GRIEVING You might start to feel emotion beginning to surface. Can you allow it to rise? You might be attuned to what it was like for you all those years earlier. Your heart might break for your younger self who had to endure the prioritization wound. Just feel for your younger self. And notice what you want to offer your younger self in this moment. Do you want to hug her? Do you want to tell him that you're so sorry he ever had to go through that? Do you want to pick them up and tell them it's going to be okay? What are you feeling compelled to do? And just notice that.

And maybe you start to notice the ways you attempted to be prioritized. Did you try to demand attention? Or give up on it altogether? Can you grieve for the you who tried to cope with this in ways that took you further away from yourself?

Be here for as long or as little feels comfortable to you. If your eyes are closed, take some time before you enter back into the room. Keep your eyes closed and bring some movement back into your fingertips, into your toes. Maybe you stretch your neck. Maybe you put your hands on your heart or your belly. Maybe you bring awareness back into your breath. Think about what you'll see when you open your eyes. Can you remember where you are?

And ever so slowly, flutter your eyes open. Take your time here.

Remember, as many times as you need, as you want. You may do this every day for a week. Or you might do it once, and come back next year, or in five years. I am so proud of you.

PIVOTING As we come to an end, I'd love for you to take a moment to acknowledge how your prioritization wound shows up today. In what ways? In what relationships? Can you finish these sentences? *If I prioritized myself, what I would change about my life right now is* _____. *If I prioritized myself, one thing I would communicate to another is* _____. For this week I'd like you to find one opportunity to prioritize yourself and to try to follow through on it. Hand on heart . . . you're doing it.

6

I WANT TO TRUST

Placing your confidence in someone else puts you in a deeply vulnerable place. When you trust, that's exactly what you're choosing to do. You are choosing to believe in others, to depend on them, and to trust that they will follow through on their words and their commitments. The first people with whom you have an opportunity to trust are almost always the people in your family. Your family teaches you about trust by what they say, what they choose, how they follow through, and what they teach you to expect from others.

Remember Natasha, the woman I spoke about at the beginning of this book who had stumbled upon her father's romantic emails with a woman who was not her mother? Natasha had seen something heartbreaking that she wasn't supposed to see, and it shattered her. The emails were a gut-wrenching betrayal of her mother, a clear rupture of the agreements and trust between her parents. But they had also broken Natasha's trust. She'd witnessed a betrayal, and then, devastatingly, been put in a position where she became *part* of the betrayal, holding her father's secret for years and keeping information from her mother that affected her mother's well-being.

Natasha had never shared this story with anyone other than me. It was a piece of information that only she and her father knew. That was a heavy burden for Natasha to carry. This broken faith stripped away a sense of trust not just in her father, but in everyone she met, especially the men she dated. It was hard for her to believe in the goodness of people. It was hard for her to believe that others would remain honest and honorable, that they'd keep their commitments and maintain their integrity. She lived her life always waiting for the other shoe to drop, anticipating that her trust would be broken yet again.

If you struggle to believe others or if you're committed to not placing your faith in others, you might have a trust wound worth exploring. Trust can be ruptured through inconsistency, lies, betrayal, and abandonment. And as we know, once trust is lost, it can feel nearly impossible to regain it and trust again.

Origins of the Trust Wound

Did you watch a parent trust freely, only to discover they'd been taken advantage of repeatedly? Did a parent, suffering from their own trust wound, tell you to watch your back or "never trust a man" or issue some other sweeping generalization that you've struggled to shake? Did you have your own experiences where the trust you freely gave was shattered in a moment, like a parent abandoning you or finding out that someone you trusted had lied or deceived you or someone you loved? When trust is broken, it can easily harden you. Walls can go up and doubt, skepticism, and suspicion tend to be ever present in your interactions and relationships.

I have found that most people really don't *want* betrayals in their past to keep them from trusting the people in their life today. They don't *want* their past experiences with duplicity or lies to keep them from believing that others can be honest, forthcoming, and trustworthy. They don't *want* to constantly scan their relationships for evidence of deceit. It's exhausting trying to live a life avoiding distrust.

Most of the clients I work with who have a trust wound ask me, "How can I learn to trust others? Is there any way that I can leave the past in the past and move forward with a clean slate?" The truth is, it can be a long, painful process to restore trust. And if lies, betrayal, or abandonment have continued beyond your childhood into your present-day romantic relationships and friendships, your lack of faith in others has probably strengthened, leaving the wound even more raw.

But all is not lost. There is a path forward, and it starts with the identification of your trust wound.

BETRAYAL

When Troy and Mark came in for their session, Troy was livid about something that had happened the night before at a party. He came into the office raging as if it had *just* occurred.

"Troy, hold on. What's going on? What happened?" I asked as I tried to slow him down.

"He did it again. He never stands up for me. He takes everyone else's side other than mine. I'm sick of it. If you can't have my back, why are you with me?" Troy was angry.

"You're not always right, Troy," Mark said quietly in response.

"But I'm not always wrong," Troy snapped back.

This wasn't the first time I had heard about this. Troy had often complained that he didn't feel like Mark had his back. He believed that his partner should always back him up and stick up for him, and felt betrayed that Mark not only didn't do this but would usually side with the other person. For his part, Mark struggled to support Troy because he didn't want to reward "bad behavior," as he termed it.

"Do you really just back someone up because they're your partner even when the way they're speaking to someone is embarrassing? Or the point they're making is not factually correct? I get that he wants my support, but it's hard to just be his cheerleader when I don't actually agree with him. Where's the line?"

Mark had a good point. Where *is* the line? But before we tried answering that question, it felt important to understand the wound at play. Troy clearly felt betrayed and didn't trust Mark to have his back. But Troy's reactivity around it suggested that this wasn't the first time in his life that he had experienced this type of betrayal.

As we dug into his family of origin, I learned that Troy's parents had divorced when he was seven and that his mom remarried a few years later. His stepfather had two of his own children, two boys, and they were close in age to Troy.

"I was the only one who got in trouble. Every single time. It didn't matter what they did, it was always my fault. My mom did nothing. She just watched as my stepdad took his sons' side constantly. They could have set me on fire and it still would have been my fault. I hated them."

Troy grew up without anyone sticking up for him. He couldn't understand how his stepfather could ignore such outrageous behavior by his own sons. Worse, his mother, the only blood relationship he had in that family, wasn't intervening on his behalf, and Troy felt betrayed that she wasn't taking a stand and protecting him. He struggled to trust that adults would do the right thing. "I get that these are your children and you're more invested in them, but how do you not only turn a blind eye to things they do, but then turn back around and place all the blame on me?"

Betrayal happens when someone breaks an explicit or implicit agreement vital to the health and well-being of the relationship. It can happen when a relational agreement is intentionally broken, like an affair or an abandonment. But it can also be felt when you need or expect something from someone—safety, protection, or prioritization—and you're left hanging. This, too, violates trust.

Betrayal can also happen through the holding back of information important for the other person to know, like failing to reveal you have been fired, you have another family, you have used a child's college savings fund to gamble, or you have been making big purchases behind your partner's back.

I see this play out in relationships often. These deceits and betrayals have a much larger impact than what some might initially think. I've had clients who make big purchases and throw away the boxes or bags before a partner can see them, and clients who send their family a substantial amount of money without communicating this to a partner. There might be explanations for this behavior, from *It's not worth the conflict* to *It's my own money and I can do with it what I please.* But whatever the explanation, it doesn't change the feeling of betrayal or the rupture in the relationship.

When there is a trust wound through betrayal, confidence is lost, and you're often left with *I can't (or don't) trust you* playing out again and again.

Betrayal can present in endless ways in a family. Can you consider if it showed up for you? Was trust broken in any way? Did you lose confidence in someone? In what ways did it teach you that others are not to be trusted?

- I felt betrayed by _____.
- The betrayal I experienced was _____.
- That has affected my ability to trust because _____.
- How I try to protect myself today is _____.

When someone you love betrays you, it can cause you to question everything in your world. Every certainty you once had, every memory you hold, is now replaced by doubt. And a life that was once filled with trust has now been robbed of that. But it is a brave and courageous act to work toward identifying the trust wound and rebuilding trust. I see you and your tender heart. You're doing it and I am cheering for you.

DECEIT

When I met Angelica, she told me that she needed to work on being able to better trust her partner. She'd been caught snooping through his phone for the umpteenth time, and he was understandably upset with her. Angelica knew she needed to stop. "I know I keep crossing a boundary of his, but it's so hard for me to trust him, even though he's never given me a reason not to."

Angelica was revealing a trust wound. She would constantly check to make sure her partner was where he said he was by following him on the Find My app, where you can track people's locations through their phone. She would search through his DMs on Instagram and look at his texts and emails to make sure he wasn't chatting with anyone she didn't know. If she stumbled upon a new name or number, she'd ask him who it was and how he knew the person. Angelica was going to great lengths to protect herself from being deceived by her partner.

I knew that there had to be an origin story that was directing this behavior. In one of our sessions Angelica shared with me that when she was twenty-one, she had found out that her aunt was actually her biological mother, and that the woman she had been calling her mom her entire life was actually her aunt. Yes, you read that correctly.

Angelica had just graduated from college, and over twenty family members attended the ceremony to support her. Afterwards, Angelica was in a bathroom stall and overheard her mom and her aunt speaking. She heard her aunt say, "Thank you so much for everything you've done for Angelica. I am so grateful that you helped me all those years ago. I wasn't ready to be a mom and she is so lucky to have you. So am I." Angelica stood there frozen in the bathroom stall. *What did she just hear? What was her aunt talking about? What did this mean?* She heard the words clearly, but her mind couldn't process the information. No one else was in the bathroom. She flushed the toilet and then stepped out. This could have been a scene from a movie. *This* was how Angelica learned that she had been deceived her entire life.

Angelica's family had kept this information about her birth story from her because they truly thought it was the right decision, but Angelica still felt deceived. She had been living a lie—and what's worse, everyone knew it except for her. This revelation sent Angelica down a path of questioning everything in her life. *Were you telling me the truth here? Were you lying to me there?* The questions kept coming.

It made sense why she felt she had to confirm everything personally, or "with her own two eyes," as she put it to me. But trusting others wasn't her only struggle. When people have been deceived, betrayed, or misguided in any way, it's easy for them to lose trust in themselves as well. *How did I not know this? How did I not see this? How could I not put two and two together? Can I not trust myself to be able to recognize things that are happening right beneath my nose?*

Can you look back at your childhood to see if there was any deceit that you either experienced or observed? Remember, deceit doesn't have to always happen *to* you for you to be affected by it. You may have watched one parent deceive another, or a parent deceive one of your siblings, and be affected by that.

- The person who was deceitful was _____.
- How that experience affected me was _____.
- How that affects me present day is _____.

ABANDONMENT

"I think she's the one." Mahmoud had just had a date the night before and he was excited to share the details with me. "I really think this could be it," he repeated. As much as I wanted to celebrate this with him, I was cautious. I had heard these exact statements multiple other times about multiple other women in the last two months alone. Mahmoud had a pattern of going on a date, hitting it off with someone, telling me he'd found his person, and then coming back the next week to tell me it was over. This cycle would repeat again and again, and today was no different.

We needed to explore further to see if we could identify what was going on. When Mahmoud was eight years old, his father told the family that he had to return to Egypt, his home country, for a work trip. He generally traveled for work once a month, but *this* time he never came back. After a couple of weeks, Mahmoud and his sisters started asking their mother when he would return. For months she would tell them that work was taking longer than he had expected, but eventually she broke the news to them that he would not be returning. He had decided to stay in Egypt.

There had been no clear answer as to why, only speculation. This abandonment was heartbreaking for the entire family. As the only boy, Mahmoud had been close to his father, and he was devastated. He had wanted to be just like his father when he grew up. Now his father was gone. *Why would Papa leave? Does he not love us? Did I do something wrong?* He couldn't make sense of what had just happened.

Childhood abandonments are a type of betrayal that happen when parents or caretakers willfully forsake or forgo their parental duties without regard for their children's overall well-being. This can happen through physical abandonment, like Mahmoud's father's departure, or it can happen through emotional abandonment, when parents struggle to be emotionally available to their child.

Did you experience abandonment growing up? By whom? What was the impact on you? And in what ways has it taught you not to trust others?

- I was abandoned by _____.
- That left me with the belief that _____.

- The way I try to protect myself today is _____.
- But what I'm realizing about that now is _____.

Coping with the Trust Wound

If you didn't feel like you could trust in your family system, it likely set you on a conscious or unconscious path of protecting yourself from betrayal, deceit, lies, and abandonment. You likely did whatever you needed to do to try to create stability and certainty for yourself. This could have been anything from looking over your shoulder or someone else's, to testing others, to closing yourself off and becoming invulnerable, to getting as close to others as quickly as possible to fabricate a sense of certainty, closeness, and commitment. But these ways of coping with a trust wound don't actually do anything to restore the trust. In fact they just maintain the distrust.

CLOSING OFF

When you've been deceived or betrayed, lied to or abandoned, it can feel like the only option is to close yourself off from others. Closing off is a way of staying protected. *If people can't get close to me, I can't be hurt.* You might choose never to share details about your life with others, to forgo real intimacy with your friends, to never date, or to limit access to yourself in any other way.

If you've ever been broken up with, you might have uttered the words *I'm never going to love again.* We say those words because the ending of a relationship is painful and is often experienced as a betrayal, and we refuse to leave ourselves vulnerable to such an experience. We never want to go through that pain again.

But this isn't reserved for relationship endings only. When someone in your family system does something that violates your trust and doesn't do anything or very little to restore it, then closing off and shutting down might feel like the only option.

The tricky thing about coping strategies is that in many ways they *do* keep you protected from the things you fear. Staying closed off may do what you want it to, but it does so at the expense of connection, closeness, intimacy, and depth in relationship. If you close off, you might be able to avoid being let down ever again, but you also never have the experience of people building trust with you, of trust being restored, and of a new story being written.

In what ways have you closed off to cope with a trust wound? In what ways has that been of service to you? Can you see the ways it has been protective in the past? But might you also notice where this coping strategy is blocking something for you today?

HYPERVIGILANCE

When the deceit Angelica's family engaged in was confirmed at her graduation, it set off a chain reaction in her. After that, she became hypervigilant with her partners, looking through their emails, texts, and DMs, living in high alert to the possible risk that she was being deceived again.

People who engage in hypervigilance are constantly scanning their environment, their relationships, and their surroundings for any indication of a lie, deception, or betrayal. This, too, is a form of self-protection. *If nothing gets by me, I can't get hurt.* It's also a lot to bear. It can feel like you're playing defense your entire life, constantly searching for where you might be deceived and betrayed. And of *course* you are. If your experience and belief are that others aren't looking out for you, that they're not to be trusted, then who's left to do that work?

I became hypervigilant during my parents' divorce. I got radically different stories from them, stories that could not possibly both be true. I knew that something was off, so I would listen very closely as the adults would speak and pick up on where someone was lying or withholding information. I'd pick up the second phone in each of their homes when I knew my parents were speaking and I'd listen in on their phone calls, just so I'd know what the *truth* was. And even though this made me good at reading people, a skill that comes in handy now, the hypervigilance robbed me of the type of joy, connection, freedom, and play I would have wanted. It's easy for this maladaptive coping strategy to make its way into adult life. It did for me. In my personal life I'd get caught tracking details or pointing out where my partner was wrong. Connor and I laughingly labeled me the "point prover," because no detail would be missed and I'd be sure to tell you about it. I can chuckle about it now, but it was a recipe for disconnection and conflict.

In what ways did you become hypervigilant to cope with a trust wound? Are you still engaging in that today? How has that been of service to you? And might you also notice where this coping strategy is affecting you negatively today?

TESTING AND SABOTAGE

When we do not trust, we often feel the need to test the people around us. You might test someone by not communicating your expectations to them. You might test them by pushing them away to see if they'll chase you and pursue you, showing you just how important you are to them. Or you might test how committed they are to you by pushing boundaries or asking for things that you know are unreasonable.

Troy didn't know if he could trust others, but he was certainly going to test them. He wanted someone to stand by his side and stick up for him. In some cases, he even knew he was in the wrong but still wanted Mark to side with him as his stepfather had with Troy's stepbrothers and as he had wanted his mother to all those years ago. "I just want to feel what it's like, you know?" Troy wanted to experience *being* the outrageous one and still have his partner back him up.

Once Troy's trust wound and origin story around betrayal had been revealed to Mark, it shifted something within the dynamic. Because we spent time tending to that wound together, Troy didn't need to test Mark as much. Trust was built intentionally, through conversation and emotional vulnerability, instead of through Troy's attempts to assess Mark by exhibiting outrageous behavior. The more the trust was established between them, the less Troy acted out in social settings.

In what ways have you tested people? Is there something that you're trying to prove through the test? And in what ways is that damaging your relationships today?

Testing can also turn into sabotage. Prior to her discovery of her father's affair, Natasha was a fully trusting girl and teenager. She had held her dad up on a pedestal. But the discovery of the emails changed everything. Overnight, Natasha came to believe that the people closest to her, the people she loved the most, were capable of unimaginable betrayal.

This is what made it hard for her to fully trust Clyde—the man she had been dating, the man who was about to propose to her—as well as all the partners who had come before him. She was waiting to discover something that had been "hidden," even though Clyde had never given her any reason not to trust him. And this distrust turned into relational sabotage.

Natasha played with the idea of ending the relationship as a form of self-protection, something she had done in all previous relationships. *If I end it before you betray me, I won't get hurt.* Natasha wouldn't have been testing Clyde; she would have been sabotaging the relationship. Natasha had a long history of finding ways to push people away, of making sure that relationships would end before she'd be devastated again.

But her sabotage and avoidance were hurting her. In this relationship, especially, Natasha had the man she wanted to marry in front of her. A man who was kind, caring, and considerate. A man who was unaware of both the struggle she was feeling at this point and the heavy burden she had carried with her for so long.

In what ways have you used sabotage as a way to protect yourself when trust is in question? What does this block you from in your present life?

ANXIOUS ATTACHMENT

Some people with a trust wound will close off and isolate themselves as adults so that they won't ever be hurt again. But others, like Mahmoud, take the opposite tack: they attach to someone very quickly, someone they haven't known for very long, in hopes of filling a void.

You might be familiar with Attachment Theory. It was first introduced to us in 1952 by the British psychoanalyst John Bowlby, and later was elaborated on by Mary Ainsworth, a developmental psychologist who conducted the famous Strange Situation study. This experiment assessed different attachment styles by observing a child's response when their mother would leave the room and then return. Securely attached babies would reconnect upon the reunion, looking for closeness and proximity with their mothers and desiring interaction. But insecurely attached babies would get angry and distressed when their mothers returned or would avoid them altogether. The Strange Situation study became a tool to measure secure and insecure attachment relationships and one we continue to utilize today as a framework for our understanding of attachment in both infancy and adulthood.

Research has shown that people who had secure attachments in infancy tend to have secure attachments in adulthood, and people who had insecure attachments in infancy tend to have insecure attachments in adulthood. When Mahmoud's father left the family, it disrupted Mahmoud's secure base. As a result, he became anxious and tried to create safety through connection, often rushing the normal pace of building a relationship and fast-forwarding right to the status of "instant boyfriend" with prospective dates. This coping strategy attempts to establish protection by getting so close to the other person so quickly that trust *can't* be violated. *If I can make this relationship stick, I won't be left again.*

Because Mahmoud was so likable, his first few dates with a new woman would go really well. There'd be a phenomenal connection. But then he'd go too far too fast. He'd start talking with those he dated about their future lives together, moving in, getting engaged and married, and the children they'd have together. At first this would come off as playful and fun, but when he pushed too hard, it became a turnoff, and the woman would decline a next date or ghost him. This happened time and again. As he said to me ruefully, "I see how it pushes people away, but I just can't break the pattern." He understood that his behavior was off-putting. He just didn't understand why he was compelled to behave this way or how to change that pattern moving forward.

"In your attempt at protecting yourself from being left, it seems like you've actually created *more* abandonment," I said.

"Whoa . . . I've never thought about it that way. I need a minute to process that."

Whether you avoid connection and intimacy to protect yourself from being abandoned again, or whether you attach quickly and anxiously in your relationships, the end result is still an absence of authentic connection. Mahmoud's relationships weren't working out because his main goal was to protect himself and ensure he'd never be left again. And that's not a great recipe for getting to know someone, forming an authentic connection, or letting a relationship naturally develop and strengthen over time. Mahmoud was unconsciously trying to force and manufacture what his father had taken from him all those years ago.

Instead of rushing connection, he would need to slow down and make himself vulnerable. He would need to create space to truly get to know someone . . . and let *that person* get to know *him*. This would always be a risk. Relationships aren't a given. There's no guarantee that a relationship will go on forever. There's no guarantee that a person will stay. And when you have a parent, a person you hope *will* be that guarantee for you, choose to up and leave you, it's a devastating experience—one that makes it nearly impossible to trust that there will be people in the world who won't abandon you.

Let's just acknowledge here that abandonment is different from an ending of relationships. This distinction is difficult for many folks to understand, especially those who have insecure attachments, and I think it's important to emphasize. People who have a trust wound centered on abandonment believe they need to find someone who will never leave them. *Promise me you won't leave. Promise me you'll stay forever.* But of course there are no guarantees. Individuals can promise it, they might say those words, but the words don't change the fear that an unresolved wound carries with it. The words don't actually establish trust.

An unresolved trust wound can wreak havoc in your present-day relationships. In addition to the pressure it puts on prospective partners, it can also draw you unconsciously to *untrustworthy* people, those who will prove your fears true. It can force you into inauthentic connections, or conversely it might cause you to avoid closeness so that you never have your heart broken again. This is no way to live. When your wounds are in control, it's impossible to establish the safety and trust that you need to head toward new beliefs, new experiences, and a place of healing.

Coping with a trust wound helps you navigate your pain in clever ways, but it doesn't do much to support the healing. Part of trusting requires you to believe in your resilience and to strengthen your discernment. It asks you to believe in your own ability to adapt and bounce back after an experience of lies, deceit, and betrayal. To learn from it. To become wiser without becoming harder and completely shutting off.

Healing the Trust Wound

Learning to trust yourself and others again is a big undertaking. Angelica was brave enough to try this with her partner. Naming and sharing her trust wound with him was the first step. Letting herself feel the depth of her family's deceit and the impact it had on her was also important. This needed to happen if she had any hope of getting to a place where she could replace her distrust with a pivot.

Eventually, instead of snooping, she would choose to share with her partner that she *wanted* to snoop because she was feeling unsure about something—and then she'd ask for clarity or assurance on that issue. Instead of tracking him on the app, she would text him and ask him where he was. Then she'd practice believing it. After all, he'd never given her a reason not to.

Once we'd identified Natasha's trust wound, she gradually came to realize that she didn't have to carry it on her own anymore. She had shared it with me, which made it a little bit lighter. And soon she would choose to share the secret with Clyde. This was a vulnerable decision, one that in itself revealed a high level of trust in Clyde. Natasha was taking a risk. She was stepping into the unknown. *The more someone knows about you, the more they can hurt you, right?* This question had rattled around in her mind for weeks.

"He'll know my most vulnerable area," she said.

"That's true," I replied. "We don't know what Clyde will do with this information. We don't know how he'll respond. But the fact that there's a part of you that's willing to share this with him tells me that some part of you believes he can hold it. That he can honor what you're telling him. It tells me that somewhere inside of you, you believe that sharing this with him will improve something for you and the relationship. If you didn't see any benefit, I don't think you'd be doing this."

The words struck a chord. Natasha had finally healed enough to step out of the role of being the keeper of her father's secret. This secret had guided her life and relationships in such significant ways, and she was ready to release herself from its control. Telling Clyde was her attempt to restore and strengthen trust instead of avoiding being hurt and engaging in sabotage.

She was fortunate to have a partner who cared deeply. When she let Clyde in and shared her secret, they became a stronger team. She successfully replaced sabotage with communication and enlisted Clyde's help in continuing to establish more trust. This was incredibly healing for Natasha. She began to replace the story she had held so close to her heart about men, about those closest to her, and about the betrayal that happens in intimate relationships. It was a beautiful process to watch.

This practice obviously works only when you have an honest partner or friend who is willing to participate in rebuilding this with you. Choosing to practice this ought to be with someone who has shown you who they are over some time, but of course you can be deceived by the people you least expect will lie to you or mislead you.

Truth is, those of us with a trust wound might always feel like it's a risk to trust someone, but there's a quote from Ernest Hemingway that gets right to the point. "The best way to find out if you can trust somebody is to trust them." This isn't meant to be a reckless act, but rather an intentional practice of trying on trust and seeing if it exists or can be built.

Part of trusting also requires you to believe in your resilience and to strengthen your discernment. It asks you to believe in your own ability to adapt and bounce back after an experience of deceit or betrayal. To learn from it. To become wiser without becoming harder and completely shutting off. This is much easier when you have a community of love and support around you to help you navigate this.

This work isn't meant to have you bypass your pain or your emotions, or to suggest that deceit and betrayal should just be overlooked. Instead, it emphasizes the value in learning that with love and support you can move through hard, awful things. In doing this, you can also tell the difference between those you can trust and those you can't, while simultaneously strengthening your trust in yourself.

I don't know if there's a way to safeguard yourself from ever being deceived, betrayed, abandoned, or misled. I believe you can minimize your exposure to it, but I'm not sure you can dodge it entirely. If you've been hurt before, you're going to do everything in your power to avoid reexperiencing the same pain. But avoiding trusting someone doesn't actually help you learn to trust again.

That's a subtle oof, so let me say it again. Avoiding trusting another doesn't actually help you learn to trust again. The only way that you can begin to trust again is by trusting through deliberate trial and error.

Establishing trust is an act of vulnerability that can feel very scary and so raw. Because it may be hard to start with trusting someone else, I often tell the people working with me to focus on building trust in themselves first. Look for any small ways you can follow through on your commitments to yourself, like going to bed when you say you're going to, drinking enough water, or moving your body on the days you commit to. See if you can build up trusting your word and your commitments and put your energy there.

If you are interested in trying out this whole "trust someone to see if you can trust them" thing, I'd love for you to think about what it is you find easy to trust about them and what it is you find hardest to trust. You can list these things for yourself to see. Notice whether the things you find hardest to trust are familiar to you or whether they feel new. Like I said before, this isn't a reckless trial and error. This is intentional and requires you to connect to your wound, share it with a person who has earned enough trust to hear it, and let that person into your inner world of doubt, suspicion, and skepticism.

I find it helps to let the person you're trying to trust more know what it is that makes it hard for you to trust. If others mock you or are insensitive or dismissive, this is a good indicator that they're not safe for you to practice this with. Also, this isn't something that you would share with someone you've just met. You want someone whose care and concern for you are felt and obvious. No matter your wound, trying to heal and repair something with someone who has little tolerance for your pain is not going to assist you in the healing. Let's try a little bit together.

- When _____ happens, it's hard for me to trust you because _____.
- This reminds me of _____, and it makes me feel _____.
- What would be helpful for me is _____.
- And what I commit to is _____.

Trust gets established through first trusting and then feeling safe in that experience. Trust happens in the brave, courageous leaps that you take when you give yourself and others the opportunity to build the trust together, when you trust and they follow through, proving to you they are trustworthy. Trust becomes much more about the present moment instead of an outcome you know nothing about in the future. Instead of *Promise me you'll never leave,* the statement shifts to *How do I feel in this moment right now?* This doesn't mean that relationships won't ever end. It doesn't mean that you won't cross a bridge with someone and then choose to go your separate ways . . . but you might be able to navigate that path with your trust still intact.

Trust isn't something that's easily reestablished. It's not something you'll claim back for yourself overnight. But it is something that you can build for yourself, as well as something that you can choose to build with others.

Origin Healing Practice

Let's take the work a bit further. If a trust wound resonated with you, let's work through the Origin Healing Practice together.

Get comfortable. You might lie down or sit on a chair. You might keep your eyes open or close them. Make sure your setting feels safe and private. As a reminder, if you're moving through trauma, it's vital you take good care. Having someone who can guide you, support you, and help create a safe space for you while you do this work is necessary.

> NAMING Can you bring into focus the first time you questioned whether you could trust someone, or the first time trust was lost? Do you remember the day? Do you remember where you were? Do you remember who put that doubt there?

> WITNESSING Now become more focused on yourself. Zoom in on the younger version of yourself who experienced the betrayal, deceit, or abandonment (remember, not the you in this moment doing the exercise). And as you watch yourself on that video, I want you to notice the feelings you were experiencing in that former moment of betrayal

and deceit. Notice what it was like to be lied to. Notice what it was like to learn that a parent had left. Notice the expression on your face and any change in your body language as sadness or disbelief start to surface. And begin to let yourself feel for that little child, younger you.

GRIEVING There's probably some emotion starting to surface by now. Can you let it surface? You might be attuned to what it must have been like for you all those years earlier. Your heart might break for your younger self who had to endure the trust wound. Feel for your younger self. And notice what you want to offer them in this moment. What do they need? Do you want to hug her? Do you want to tell him that you're so sorry he was betrayed? Do you want to pick them up and tell them that you know how painful the deceit was? What are you feeling compelled to do? And just notice that.

Be here for as long or as little feels comfortable to you. If your eyes are closed, take some time before you enter back into the room. Keep your eyes closed and bring some movement back into your fingertips, into your toes. Maybe you stretch your neck. Maybe you put your hands on your heart or your belly. Maybe you bring awareness back into your breath. Think about what you'll see when you open your eyes. Can you remember where you are? And ever so slowly, flutter your eyes open. Take your time here.

Remember, as many times as you need, as you want. You may do this every day for a week. Or you might do it once, and come back next year, or in five years. I am so proud of you.

PIVOTING As we come to an end, I'd love for you to take a moment to acknowledge how your trust wound shows up today. In what ways? In what relationships? Can you finish this sentence? *If I allowed myself to fully trust, if I wasn't afraid to just be, what would be different is* _____. For this week I'd like you to see if you can just notice when there would be an opportunity to replace an old way with a new way.

WRITING YOUR TRUST WOUND A LETTER

Here's one last exercise for your trust wound Origin Healing Practice. I find letter writing to be incredibly powerful. It's a place where you can be fully expressed and also put into words what it is you're reclaiming. If you have a trust wound, I highly encourage you to make time to do this.

I'd like you to write a letter to your trust wound (yes, this letter will start "Dear Trust Wound"). This letter ought to have compassion for the wound, and it might have gratitude for the ways your wound has tried to cope. But I also want you to tell it what it is you'd like to claim back for yourself. What do you want it to know about you? What do you want it to know about where you are in your life right now? What do you want to be in charge of instead of letting it be in charge? Speak directly to it. Begin to have more of a relationship with it. Part of healing a trust wound requires the wound itself to trust *you*. Let it know what it can trust from you.

Again, this work doesn't happen overnight. You might come back to this letter over and over again. You might add to it. You might write to your trust wound many times. But for now, just begin.

7

I WANT TO FEEL SAFE

As a child, you relied heavily on your parents and caretakers for safety. Your parents are meant to protect, respect, be attuned to, advocate for, and set rules and boundaries to maintain your safety. But as we know, the adults in our lives don't always get it right. In fact, sometimes they're the ones missing the signs, doing the harm, or being reckless with our lives, putting us in harm's way.

Certainly there are no guarantees that from the beginning of your life you will be treated with care and protected from harm. This *should* be your experience. You *should* have safety within your family. Your home *should* be the place that you can go for comfort, security, peace, stability, and predictability. Home *should* be where you go to retreat when the world around you is scary, threatening, and hard. (I don't use the word *should* often, but now feels like the appropriate time to employ it.)

Of course, your parents can't protect you from everything out there, but when members of your own family are abusive, negligent, exploitative, domineering, reckless, or emotionally immature, it's quite easy for a safety wound to be born. You know that saying "Home is where the heart is"? Well, that's not true for everyone. Home isn't a place that everyone wants to return to. Sometimes home is where the

157

unpredictability is. Sometimes home is where the chaos is. And sometimes home is where the abuse is.

Origins of the Safety Wound

When we talk about safety, the conversation must include abuse. I share this up front with you because I want you to take good care of yourself as you continue reading this chapter. Whether you have ever experienced or witnessed abuse or not, reading about it can be triggering, emotional, and overwhelming. I am asking you to be a good gauge for yourself as you move through these pages.

ABUSE

Abuse, without question, creates a safety wound. When abuse is present, safety is absent. Full stop. And when that abuse happens in your own home or the people in your home don't stop it from happening, you experience a major betrayal and loss of trust originating from your family. As the author, professor, and activist bell hooks so aptly puts it in *All About Love*: "Abuse and neglect negate love. Care and affirmation, the opposite of abuse and humiliation, are the foundation of love. It is a testimony to the failure of loving practice that abuse is happening in the first place." Love and abuse cannot coexist.

We're going to look at abuse through the lens of family systems, but you might identify something that rings true at this very point in your adult life. If you are in an abusive relationship, you can call the National Domestic Violence Hotline at 1-800-799-SAFE (7233) or visit domesticshelters.org to access professional help. Below I will outline different types of abuse and what they could have looked like in your childhood. Please take care.

Abuse is defined as a pattern of behavior used by one person to gain and maintain power and control over another. There are six types of abuse: physical, sexual, verbal/emotional, mental/psychological, financial/economic, and cultural/racial/identity. All forms of abuse utilize the power and control that one person has over another, and it's why children are highly susceptible to abuse, given the power and control dynamics already embedded in the adult-child relationship.

You're probably familiar with what most of these types of abuse are, but I think it's important for us to take a closer look together.

Physical abuse threatens a child's physical safety. Maybe you watched one parent physically abuse the other parent or one of your siblings and you felt helpless, scared, and unsafe. Maybe you were the target of the physical abuse, the recipient of a parent's anger and re-activity. Maybe they would throw things at you, punch, hit, kick, or strangle you. There are endless gut-wrenching stories of children living in fear waiting for the abuse to come their way. I've had clients share stories about how parents would put their cigarettes out on them, or parents who would throw heavy objects at their head. One client even told me that his father made his brother who had cerebral palsy jump up onto the sofa and down off it as a form of punishment.

But physical abuse can happen even if there's no physical touch. It can look like an adult becoming physically threatening and intimidating. Like someone who chases after you even if they don't catch you, or a parent who stands in front of your bedroom door so you can't leave. You may have felt scared physically for your safety or felt trapped or intimidated in your physical space.

Sexual abuse threatens a child's sexual safety. About one in ten children will be sexually abused before their eighteenth birthday. But because childhood sexual abuse often goes unreported, we know that the numbers could be quite a bit higher. You may have been sexually abused by someone in your home, like a parent, stepparent, sibling, or cousin. Your abuser may have threatened to hurt you or someone you love to make sure you wouldn't tell anyone, they may have convinced you that you deserved what was happening, or they may have told you that what was happening was acceptable and normal. You may have been afraid, or you may have felt confused, recognizing that something was off but experiencing sexual pleasure nonetheless. I've had clients share with me how uncomfortable it was to be exposed to pornography at such an early age or to have a stepparent speak to them in a sexual manner when no one else was around. Child sexual abuse involves touch, and it also involves noncontact sexual acts between an adult and a minor or between minors when one minor exerts power and control over the other.

Verbal and emotional abuse is any verbal or emotional attempt to scare, isolate, control, or degrade you. Earlier in this book I mentioned statements of harm. Verbal and emotional abuse can happen through nitpicking, engaging in character assassination, insulting your appearance or accomplishments, embarrassing you publicly, or being patronizing. Words cut so deep. One of my clients shared with me how his stepfather, who coached his hockey team when he was growing up, would constantly comment about what a terrible athlete he was in front of his teammates. One day in front of everyone he said to him, "Your mother really made a mistake by letting your father get her pregnant. She should have made him pull out." This comment was downright abusive and degrading, both to my client and his mother.

Mental and psychological abuse falls under the category of emotional abuse, but it's a bit more nuanced. Abusers use psychological abuse to control, terrorize, and denigrate their victims. A parent might have repeatedly threatened to harm you, themselves, or someone else. They may have harshly blamed you for anything and everything that went wrong. They may have threatened to abandon you if you weren't well behaved, given you the silent treatment and ignored you for long periods of time, or made you feel crazy by moving things around or hiding things that you needed for school or self-care. A client of mine shared with me that when her father was angry with her, he would find projects or homework she had been working on and threaten to rip them up or destroy them. He'd take her favorite clothing and threaten to ruin it in front of her unless she did what he said. Another client of mine said that when he came out to his parents, his father stopped speaking to him for years. At that point in his life my client kept a journal, and he found that any sheet of paper that mentioned his being gay would be ripped out of it.

Financial and economic abuse is an attempt to control a victim with money. Although you might generally think about this type of abuse played out between adults, it happens between parent and child as well. Your parent might have prevented you from having access to the money you'd saved from birthdays or gifts over the years. They might have stolen from you, or maybe they put credit cards, bills, or bank accounts in your name without your knowledge. They may have exploited you for money or punished you for spending money of your own.

Cultural/racial/identity abuse happens when an abuser uses aspects of your culture, race, and identity to inflict pain and suffering and to control you. This might play out in a family where there are differences in culture and race, possibly through a stepparent dynamic or in an adoptive or fostering dynamic. Maybe you heard cultural or racial slurs growing up, or you were threatened to be outed by someone in your family. Or you may have observed particular dietary or dress customs because of your faith and were ridiculed or denied what was necessary for you to honor that. An Indian client shared with me that after her parents got divorced, her mother remarried a white man; he would make comments about how much hair she had on her arms and face. He'd make fun of her and tell her she'd better shave because otherwise people at school might mistake her for an animal. It was disgusting and degrading.

There are two other forms of abuse I want to acknowledge: neglect and exploitation. Neglect involves the lack of proper food, clothing, shelter, medical care, and supervision. Neglect can happen either actively, with intent, or passively, without intent. A parent might fail to tend to your medical, hygienic, or nutrition needs. Your parents may have left you at home without any proper care or supervision. Or they may have ignored you when you came to them with emotional or physical needs, causing emotional distress and agony.

Exploitation of a child is the act of using a child for profit, labor, sexual gratification, or some other personal or financial advantage. A child is usually given something in exchange, like gifts, money, drugs, affection, or status. This could look like someone in your life prostituting you or trafficking you for their personal gain, or it could look like an authority figure using you to hold, sell, or transport drugs for them.

Okay. Big breath. That was a lot. If you experienced any of the above, whether you're identifying it right now for the first time or you've known for a long time, I recommend working with a licensed therapist to provide support in processing the abuse. There are safe spaces for you to do this very important work.

RECKLESSNESS

For some, a safety wound develops when parents know or ought to know that their conduct, behavior, decisions, and choices will likely cause harm, but they consciously disregard the substantial and unjustifiable risk anyway. Recklessness could look like a parent who's intoxicated driving their child, or parents who have their child in the car with them when they go pick up their drugs. It could be parents whose addiction puts their children at risk, like leaving the oven on because they passed out or leaving their used needles or drugs out in the open. Recklessness leaves children feeling unsafe, exposed, and vulnerable to harm.

Amir came to therapy because his spending was out of hand. He shared with me that he would buy designer clothes and shoes all the time, drop money on trips and hotels, and indulge in any luxury experience he could give himself and his friends. He made great money, but he revealed to me that he spent every last dollar he had. He was embarrassed that at forty-nine he had no savings.

"Like, zero. I don't have money saved away. It comes in and it goes out. I keep up the image because I spend constantly. I think people think I'm wealthy, but that's not true. I haven't accrued any wealth. I make boatloads of money and then spend boatloads of money like it's my second job. I'm so pathetic."

Amir was fed up with himself. He had been behaving this way for a long time. He had a stable job that he had been at for close to twenty years, but he had not been financially wise. He didn't own any assets and was even starting to accrue some debt.

"I need your help. Why am I doing this?" he asked.

This wasn't a case of someone just scraping by and living paycheck to paycheck. Amir was a financially privileged man who was setting himself up for a scary and unnecessarily stressful future. He was consciously disregarding the many risks that came along with spending everything he made. It was reckless behavior. I wondered if there might be a safety wound at the heart of these dodgy actions.

When we dove into his childhood, Amir shared with me that his father was quick to rage. When I asked him how that would look and play out, he said that it always happened when his father would drive him places.

"Everyone thought my dad was this gentle giant, but when he and I were alone in the car, he would become enraged and drive the car so fast. I'm talking like eighty to ninety miles an hour in a thirty-five zone. And then he would slam on the brakes and do it again. I would beg him to stop. I'd cry and tell him I was scared. But it didn't matter. He wanted to make me scared. He wanted me to fear for my life. He liked feeling in control and I never understood why. He would pick me up from school every day because my mom didn't drive, and this is what he would do when he was mad. He didn't even need to be angry at me. He could have been pissed at my mom, at our neighbor, at his brother. It didn't matter."

Amir was breathing heavily after sharing this with me. It was up-setting to remember it, but he had more to say. "Why did my life not matter to him?" he exclaimed in disbelief. "Why did it not matter to him if he got us killed or hurt me?"

Amir was identifying a safety wound in the form of his father's recklessness with him. For you, it might have been that your parents left their loaded gun out where you could reach it, or a parent who left drugs out on a table that you could access. As we continued our work together, Amir started to see how he was carrying forward his father's recklessness into his own life. It was just disguised a bit differently. Amir had come to believe that his life didn't matter to his dad or his mom, who had never stepped in. *If it doesn't matter to them, why should it matter to me?*

Amir began to live recklessly. He loved taking physical risks in his twenties—participating in extreme sports, partying hard—but he normalized it by calling himself an adrenaline junkie. As he grew older, he found a new way to live on the edge: financial irresponsibil-ity. But what remained true throughout was the message that he kept receiving and offering himself: *Your safety doesn't matter.* Amir didn't know how to care about himself. He didn't know how to send himself the message that his life, his well-being, his current and future safety were a priority.

It's not easy to make a shift toward safety when your past com-municates to you that your safety isn't a priority. And it can be espe-cially hard to make that adjustment when a safety origin wound comes at the hands of a parent.

Can you look back at your childhood and see if anyone in your family system was ever reckless with you? Let's explore a little together.

- The person who was reckless with my life was _____.
- What I remember about that experience was _____.
- How that affects me present day is _____.

DISSOCIATION

Dissociation is a mental process of disconnecting from one's own body and thoughts. It's often described as an experience in which people separate entirely from themselves, as if their mind has been transported elsewhere even though their body is still in front of you. And although there are adaptive dissociative experiences, a maladaptive dissociative experience disconnects you from yourself. Dr. Bessel van der Kolk, an expert on trauma and the author of *The Body Keeps the Score,* explains dissociation as the process of "simultaneously knowing and not knowing." Dissociation can happen in response to unprocessed trauma, and if you've ever encountered someone in a dissociated state, you know how scary the experience can be—especially for a child who likely doesn't understand what's happening.

A child might worry about their parent because of how checked out they seem. They might feel scared about why a parent can't remember important details, or they might feel physically unsafe if a parent becomes dissociated while in conversation, while driving, or while cooking.

My client Tony had shared that it was hard for him to get close to people. He had been single his entire adult life and was resistant to going on dates. His friends urged him to go to therapy to try to figure out why. We spent time learning about his family of origin and what it was like for him growing up. After a few sessions, Tony shared with me that his father had become physically abusive toward his mother. The abuse started when Tony was about nine years old and was something that would happen often. Although Tony never saw it, he watched his mother become a shell of herself.

"It was like she was there, but she wasn't. It was like she was off in the distance but there was no way to bring her back. She was the best mother I could have ever asked for before all of this." It was scary for Tony to watch her slowly deteriorate. He never felt safe in that home and worried that one day his father would come for him, too.

Tony begged his father to stop, but it wasn't until he was big enough and strong enough to go toe-to-toe with his father that he could put an end to it. "I knocked him out and he never touched her again."

Tony was glad that the abuse stopped, but it didn't bring his mom back. She remained a shell of herself. This was such a devastating loss. He had really needed her and was angry that his father had not only robbed his mother of her old personality but had also robbed Tony of the mother who had once so loved and cared for her only son.

Tony feared that love and connection would inevitably be lost in relationships. Relationships for him were a place where one felt unsafe, where people detached and psychologically disappeared. Instead of risking the unbearable pain again, he had chosen to disconnect from dating and love altogether. Tony was afraid of losing people. He was afraid of being loved and then having it ripped away. It had been too much for his system to process, so he hid from love. This was a powerful starting point for us as Tony began his work around healing his safety wound and reclaiming safety for himself so that he could make room for love in his life.

Can you look back at your childhood and see if anyone in your family system was ever dissociated? And how did that experience affect safety for you?

- The person who was dissociated was _____.
- What I remember about that experience is _____.
- What was scary about that for me was _____.
- How that affects me present day is _____.

SCARY SITUATIONS

Many safety wounds come from abusive situations. Parents, stepparents, caretakers, adults, or older siblings can be reckless, domineering, negligent, and abusive in obvious and subtle ways. But I would be doing us a disservice if I didn't acknowledge that a safety wound can surface in a family even when there is no power, control, recklessness, neglect, or exploitation at play.

Sometimes an absence of safety becomes obvious even when parents are doing their best, such as a parent living with money scarcity that a child is only too aware of. A child's basic needs can be taken care of, but the child might still worry about the parent's wellbeing. Children of divorced parents, both of whom are doing their absolute best to co-parent gracefully, can still feel afraid to share that they had a good time with the other parent during their weekend away. And sometimes the absence of safety is created because the unimaginable happens—like losing a parent—leaving the child fearing other worst-case scenarios (that the other parent might die, too).

The above examples are scenarios where there is no power or control at play. Parents aren't gaining something by engaging with their children in this way. Parents can do everything right, and there *still* might be a safety wound that gets created.

Aaliyah's safety wound originated one evening when she was a little girl. Her parents were out to dinner, leaving her in the care of her grandmother, and her grandmother had a massive stroke. Aaliyah shared how, despite being only nine years old, she held her grandmother's head to try to stabilize her, called 911, and assisted the medics when they arrived. Her grandmother recovered, but this event was so scary and shocking that Aaliyah never wanted to be home alone ever again.

In her adult life, Aaliyah had successfully avoided living alone. She was perpetually partnered; I'm talking serial monogamy with no days off between partners. She wasn't proud of her behavior, but when something was ending with one guy, she would start up something new with another (her "backup plan") so that she could transition to living with that person. Despite her romantic history, she said she had never actually cared deeply for someone, and she reported that her behavior in relationships was a source of deep shame for her. The question was why.

As we explored further, Aaliyah began to see how the safety wound that originated with her grandmother's scary situation led her to prioritize cohabitation over connection. This urge pushed her into relationships in which what *she* wanted, desired, or cared for in a partner couldn't matter; her focus was on "sealing the deal" and fast-forwarding to immediately living together. She had never slowed down to even consider what was important for her in partnership, and she stayed in relationships that weren't good for her to avoid having to live alone.

I remember her jaw dropping the moment we connected the safety wound dots. She had a lightbulb moment and everything changed for her. This pattern wasn't about making reckless decisions; her behavior was in fact an attempt at creating safety for herself. If she had a boyfriend on call, she wouldn't be alone to deal with scary situations like the one that happened to her grandmother. Her self-criticism changed to self-compassion . . . with a big side of ownership.

Did you ever experience an absence of safety growing up where control or power dynamics were not at play? What happened that wasn't anyone's fault but still left you feeling unsafe?

- One thing I was scared of growing up that was no one's fault was _____.
- How that's affected me throughout my life is _____.
- What this gets in the way of present day is _____.

Coping with the Safety Wound

Living in a home environment where safety was lacking took something from you. It changed you. But the ways you responded to feeling unsafe growing up don't have to be the ways in which you live today.

Of course it's a scary world and not everyone you meet is safe. But part of your work is to be able to feel the difference between those who are a threat and those who aren't. It's a muscle you want to strengthen. I know that there are people out there who do cause pain, but there are also people out there who want to be a safe haven and a secure base for you. I know it can be hard to trust, but let's see if there's a way to start taking the tiniest of steps in that direction.

LIVING IN FEAR

So many children live in fear. Some live in fear of their physical safety, while others live in fear of disappointing their parents. They worry about sharing their emotions with their caretakers and being reprimanded for it or setting boundaries and being ridiculed and shamed. In unsafe familial environments, living in fear might mean you're afraid of how a person will react, respond, judge, shame, mock, and override you.

This might bring a lot to the surface for you. Maybe you've thought about the ways you lived in fear growing up, but when I met Miyako and Jin, neither had ever considered or even known to look at their origin wounds.

Miyako and Jin were both in their mid-thirties. The two had been together for four years, and Miyako was eager for an engagement. Jin was turned off by what he perceived as Miyako's ultimatums, and I got the sense her demands seemed to be pushing him in the opposite direction. Miyako didn't see them as ultimatums, however. She saw them as setting a boundary. They both wanted children, they loved each other, and they had similar visions for life, but if he wasn't going to move forward with her, she felt she needed to move on with her life.

I soon learned that Miyako had been communicating this ultimatum/boundary for an entire year. Five other deadlines that year alone: Valentine's Day, her birthday, his birthday, a Parisian trip they had taken where she dreamed of being proposed to in front of the Eiffel Tower, and Thanksgiving. Each came and went without a proposal. This was devastating for Miyako. She'd pack her bags and go stay with a friend for a few nights, start looking at new apartments, and have a breakup conversation with Jin, but ultimately she'd always come back and want to try again. This time she promised was the last.

I soon learned that Miyako had lost her job about a year prior. She shared how difficult this had been for her. It was a dream job and she had been let go because she wasn't performing up to the expectations the company had of her. This was a devastating blow for Miyako. She was so embarrassed by this that she hid it from everyone other than Jin. Instead of looking for a new job, she had remained jobless for an entire year, pretending that she was still at the same gig. But behind closed doors she was struggling. She'd cry every night to Jin when he'd return from work, and she'd look to him for emotional support. She needed validation and encouragement from him almost nightly.

"How has this affected you, Jin?" I asked.

"I'm happy to support her. We all go through hard things, but it's been a while. How long is she going to go without working? How long is she going to keep pretending? Plus, it puts me in an awkward position keeping up the facade that she's still working there."

Miyako reacted quickly. "Is this why you don't want to marry me? Is this why you're avoiding an engagement?"

Jin didn't have the answer right in that moment, but he knew he wasn't quite certain about marriage yet. He was stressed about her job situation and eventually admitted that he would delay coming home at night. "It's just a lot to come home every night and listen to the same stuff. You're struggling, I get it, but you're not getting any help or doing anything about it. You just want me to help and I'm tired. It's exhausting for me, and it does create some concerns for me."

It was clear to me that Jin was having a reaction to being cast in the role of emotional supporter. When I asked him about his parents, what their relationship was like, he carefully responded that they respected each other. They weren't in love. They simply coexisted, not asking much of each other, but they took care of his sister and Jin himself. I then asked him to tell me about his mom.

"She was a quiet woman, but she was really hardworking and instilled a good work ethic in me."

Miyako quietly interjected, "Can you tell her about the suicide stuff, Jin?"

I sat in silence with them as Jin decided whether he was ready to share something personal with me.

Jin looked up at me. He needed to find some safety in my face. I smiled and nodded, suggesting that I could hold whatever it was he would share.

"I was thirteen when my mom first threatened suicide. She wasn't well. She was really unhappy with her life and the relationship she had with my dad. But the moment I became a teenager, she started sharing things with me that weren't appropriate. I feel like she thought that because I was a teenager I wasn't a kid anymore, or something like that, and she would just dump things on me because she thought I could handle it." He took a moment to collect himself.

"So, yeah, she would threaten suicide often. Every few weeks. And it wasn't just the contemplation of it. She would share this with me when she was upset and say her goodbyes to me. And then I would have to cry and scream and beg and plead and stay with her to make sure she didn't do anything. And she never did. Not once did she actually attempt it, but she threatened it over and over and over again for years."

I could see Miyako squeezing Jin's hand tighter. His head dropped and he began to cry.

"That must have been so scary for you, Jin. Just so frightening. To constantly fear for your mother's life and to also feel the weight of having to be the one to save her each time."

He nodded.

Home wasn't a safe environment for Jin. It was an environment that asked him to step into the inappropriate role of emotional care-taker for his mom. He had to be on high alert constantly, and he had to be available whenever she would need him. If you've ever watched someone you love live with immense pain, you know how terrible it is to witness. Jin loved his mom so much and wanted her to be okay, but this was a role he should never have found himself in. Jin lived in fear constantly as a child. No one knew that this was going on, and he was too scared and embarrassed to speak of it with anyone else.

We spent some time in silence, acknowledged the raw feelings in the room, and explored what Jin would need once they left the session. Jin had just named a safety wound. He was beginning to see just how unsafe he had been in his home. He couldn't trust his father to step in and take some responsibility, and he couldn't trust his mother to get the support and care she needed to keep herself safe. The repeated threats created in Jin a deep fear that his mother would hurt herself and he would feel personally responsible for not being able to stop her. Jin had experienced a type of abuse he had never fully identified, and it was the missing piece in understanding his resistance to proposing to and marrying Miyako.

Even though Miyako and Jin's mom were different, they had some traits in common. Jin was afraid of having to serve as the only emotional support in Miyako's life, just as he'd done for his mom. And he was concerned that Miyako wasn't getting the help and support she needed to move through this tough time, an experience he knew all too well.

When your home environment requires you to be on the lookout for yourself or for others, it's nearly impossible for you to feel safe. You'll find it hard to connect to ease, peace, joy, or pleasure. You're either in anticipation mode or in protection mode, and neither one lets you rest, restore, relax, or feel free. Instead, you're always on high alert, waiting for the next threat to make its way to you. Maybe the signal was a beer can being opened or your mom's departure to go work her night shift, leaving you at home alone with your abusive stepparent. Maybe the alert was the yelling you heard downstairs or the very specific eyebrow raise your father would give. What was the trigger that moved home from safe to unsafe for you?

Home ought to be where you can rest. It ought to be where you can take off the armor, regroup, and restore. But for so many, home is not a place of rest, and sadly, for most children or adults with safety wounds, it was where they felt the most afraid and alone.

SHUTTING DOWN

Threats, unresolved anger, unwarranted and unwanted accusations, cutting comments, and anxiety-inducing experiences are things so many children are expected to just brush off or ignore, but all of these can be incredibly threatening and uncomfortable, leaving their home environment feeling unsafe.

Maybe you had a parent who always commented about your looks and your appearance, making you feel so uncomfortable that you started wearing baggy clothes that covered your entire body. Maybe your parents fought constantly, and the yelling and noise never made you feel safe at home. Or maybe it was your mother's or father's incessant sense of panic that made you feel like something terrible was always about to happen.

These experiences can rob you of the space to be, to feel, to express, and to emote. The response is often to shut down instead of opening to the pain you're feeling.

I remember when we started our therapy together. Ally sat down on the sofa and said, "It's time."

"It's time for what?" I asked.

"I need to learn how to tell people what I'm feeling. It's so hard for me, and if I don't figure this out, I'm never going to be able to keep a partner."

Ally was a twenty-five-year-old young professional living in New York City. Her girlfriend had just broken up with her, but this breakup was more of a trend than a singular event. Ally had confessed that she had never broken up with anyone in her life. "People always leave me. And they always leave me because they say I'm not vulnerable enough."

I could tell that Ally was annoyed by this. She agreed with the feedback from her exes, but she didn't like it.

"What about the feedback makes you uncomfortable?" I asked.

"I guess because it means I have to become vulnerable, right? If people leave me because I don't share myself with them, then I guess I need to start doing that."

"That's true," I said. "But I wonder if instead of brute-forcing yourself to become vulnerable, we instead get more curious about why vulnerability is tough for you in the first place?"

Ally's resistance was our neon sign. It was the hint that a wound was nearby, and we'd need to venture toward it together.

"What's the first thing you think of when I say the word *vulnerable*?" I asked.

"Sharing myself?" she answered tentatively.

"Great," I said. "So can you tell me about your experience of sharing yourself growing up with your family?"

Ally was revealing to me that vulnerability didn't feel safe. She struggled with it, and even though she had gotten the same feedback from multiple exes, it was still hard for her to override the part of herself that didn't want to share. Shutting down and not sharing herself kept her safe from something, even though it created its own lack of safety: the ending of relationships. Whatever that something was, it was more important or powerful than maintaining these relationships. Her protection mode was in full force, and I knew it had to be for a good reason.

Ally eventually shared with me a devastating story. "When I was either twelve or thirteen, I remember it all starting. We would all sit down to dinner together—my mom, my dad, and me—and my dad would ask me how school was or how I was doing or just anything about what was going on in my life, and one day when I started to answer his question, it was as if my mom had some kind of mental break. She screamed at me and said, 'Stop flirting with my husband!' Then she stood up and stormed away. My dad and I stared at each other and had no idea what had happened. It was unreal. I know my dad talked to her about it, but I was never given an apology, nothing was acknowledged, and it kept happening for a few weeks. Every evening my mom would make comments under her breath about me at dinner. If my dad asked me a question or showed any interest in my life, she would make these terrible comments about me flirting, or she'd say that she couldn't believe that I would be attracted to him."

This was an incredibly painful story to hear, one that was deeply disturbing. Ally's mom was technically experiencing a psychotic episode, confusing what was real and what wasn't. And although Ally and her father knew something was off, the severity of the mental health challenges went unaddressed.

I had asked Ally whether she knew anything about her mother's past and history. She shared that her mother had experienced sexual abuse when she was a teenager and that it was unresolved. "I know my mom never worked it out. She just shut down and never discussed it, never processed it. It's awful. I can't imagine what she went through, but her pain and trauma was just being poured onto me and that wasn't right."

Because Ally's mother had been abused when she herself was thirteen, it seemed that she went on high alert when Ally turned the same age. Her accusations seemed to be her way of looking for any sexual misconduct. We never had Ally's mom in therapy with us, but we questioned whether she was projecting her own self-blame onto Ally. Did Ally's mom feel responsible for the abuse she endured? Was she blaming Ally for things that weren't actually happening because her trauma was unresolved? These were questions that Ally considered.

You can see how pain can pass from generation to generation, and how unaddressed mental health challenges can wreak havoc in a family. Even though there was no sexual abuse going on in Ally's life, the sexual abuse her mother had endured from the past was dominating the family, leaving Ally feeling unsafe. Ally's mother's anger, her unresolved trauma, and the unwarranted accusations against Ally were ever present. Ally eventually stopped engaging even after the accusations had ceased. "I found every reason under the sun not to have to sit down for dinner with them and to be out of the house as much as possible. I could feel her staring at me, and I could feel her anger toward me constantly. And my dad really didn't do anything about it. He'd just tell me not to worry about it. So I learned to shut down. I didn't understand why my mom hated me so much at the time. It wasn't until later that I learned more about her past and some of this started to make more sense to me."

Ally shook her head. "Is this why you think I struggle to be vulnerable?"

This story was hard to hear, as I envisioned a young girl having to combat and dodge those emotional bullets. But I couldn't help but smile as Ally found her origin wound. "Ally, I think you're connecting some dots all on your own."

There was no room for Ally to just be, to share anything about her day, or to have normal and appropriate conversations with either of her parents. She learned quickly that opening up and sharing weren't safe because of the daily attacks from her mother. Safety, Ally learned, was staying closed off, distracting herself, busying herself, and disconnecting from her parents as much as possible. She became hypervigilant, never looking at her dad, never taking a seat next to him at family outings or events, and never asking him questions when her mom was around. Ally had cracked the code. She found a way to protect herself, but it required her to quiet herself, close off, and not share anything.

Of course Ally's story, like those of all of my clients, is unique and personal. You may not have had a parent with the kind of trauma in her background that Ally's mom had or who transferred their pain in the exact same way. But you may have had a parent who couldn't handle when you were sad or would cry. Or parents who would react strongly if you weren't the "perfect child" they expected you to be. Maybe you had parents who pressured you to agree with their beliefs, or gave you attention only when you dressed a certain way or wore your hair a certain way. Or maybe you had a parent who would tell you repeatedly that you should be more like your sibling.

No wonder children shut down or learn that it's unsafe to share themselves fully. No wonder those children become adults who struggle to open up or adults who overshare with people who haven't earned the right to hear their vulnerability.

If it's hard for you to open up and share yourself with others, perhaps consider whether a safety wound is at play. Just take a moment to tune into your story and your life. What do you believe will happen if you share your thoughts, emotions, and feelings with others? Do you feel comfortable sharing only certain things? Do you struggle to disagree or express an alternative opinion? And if you look back, can you find anything or anyone in your family of origin that made your freedom of expression challenging?

Ally saw how her safety wound was keeping her from opening up to the important people in her life. This wound from the past was robbing her of the connection, presence, commitment, and joy she craved from her relationships. Maybe that's true for you, too. As you keep yourself protected and safe, might you also be cutting yourself off from the people who could care about you, who could love you, and who would safely want to hear about your life and what's going on in your inner world?

Healing the Safety Wound

When you're a child who can't trust others to prioritize your safety, you will adapt in the ways you need to in order to survive. It's no wonder that children with a safety wound can easily grow up to be adults who struggle to trust others, trust themselves, or work tirelessly at creating some type of safety for themselves that can easily get in the way of the type of connection, closeness, and intimacy they might crave.

Amir, Tony, Aaliyah, Miyako and Jin, and Ally were all doing their best, but the way they were creating safety for themselves was creating disconnection in their lives. When you protect the wound at all costs, you leave it unhealed. The protection one gains usually comes at the expense of other important goals in one's life: partnership, connection, closeness, and intimacy.

Healing the safety wound is complicated. As you've seen all along, part of healing requires being able to share your story, something that everyone in this book has leaned into. But part of sharing your story also requires there to be trust between the person sharing and the person receiving. That's why therapy can be such a beautiful space for someone to start. That relationship between client and therapist is a sacred one. And it's why so many people who have endured such terrible things in their life choose to start there, to practice opening up, sharing, and being witnessed and honored by another human.

It can be in that experience where you can begin to *feel* what it is like to truly be safe. As Dr. Alexandra Solomon says, "Trust and trauma unfortunately go hand in hand." Meaning that if you're going to begin to heal trauma, it will ask you to trust, the very thing that was shattered for you when your safety was not upheld. A bold and brave decision.

Amir, Tony, Aaliyah, Miyako and Jin, and Ally had something in common. They all had a relationship with me that was safe enough for them to begin revealing their story. Miyako and Jin had each other, too. A loving relationship dynamic, which can be found in partnership, in therapy, in friendship, and beyond, is a powerful healing force. This work can be difficult to do alone, and it's why a relational healing process is something I encourage.

If you are looking for something to work on alone, I encourage trying a mindfulness practice. I've included one below. When it comes to creating safety for yourself, so much of the work requires you to *show* your body what safety is instead of trying to *think* about what safety is or trying to *tell* yourself what it is. *Embodied self-regulation,* a term coined by psychologist Catherine Cook-Cottone, is the experience of regulating the self and our emotions through mindfulness practices instead of just processing them intellectually. It supports you in being able to *feel* when you can trust that you are safe and when you're not.

I should mention here that if you do have trauma, mindfulness practices can feel particularly challenging and uncomfortable. Please know that this is not uncommon. Don't push yourself; listen to your body. It's also especially important for you take your time and establish the necessary safety when healing trauma that originated from a safety wound and to work with trauma-informed professionals on your healing path. I appreciate how Dr. Gabor Maté describes trauma. He maintains that "trauma is not what happens *to* you, it is what happens *in* you, as a result of what happened to you."

To connect with yourself and to connect with others in and of itself is healing. What a profound experience to begin to write a new story of safety. What a profound experience to be able to find safety within yourself and safety within your chosen relationships. This is a goal worth working toward. This is the beautiful work that you come back to again and again.

Origin Healing Practice

The Origin Healing Practice you learned in previous chapters is also available to you here, as well: naming, witnessing, grieving, and pivoting to new behaviors. But because there's a high likelihood that your trauma might be sitting next to you, I'm going to ask you to take very good care of yourself in this instance. You may want to skip over the Origin Healing Practice entirely here, or wait until you can do it alongside a trauma-informed therapist so you have proper care and support.

Instead, I have provided a guided meditation designed to help you experience safety in your body.

ORIGIN HEALING EXERCISE: A GUIDED MEDITATION

This exercise is designed for you to practice *feeling* what safety is like in your body instead of trying to *think* about what safety is.

Find a comfortable, calm place in your home, ideally one with privacy. Sit in a relaxed pose. I generally recommend keeping your eyes closed, but if it feels safer to keep your eyes open, do that. Let your spine be strong, maintaining your posture while the front of your body is soft, open, and supple. Let yourself feel the strength in your back and softness in your front.

Now make contact with your breath. Be aware of it dropping into the body and falling out. There's no need to force it. Simply allow yourself to observe the wave of the breath falling in and dropping out. As you do this, bring your attention and awareness to your eyebrows and eyelids, letting them soften. Find ease and softness in your face, letting the muscles of your face become supple and slack. Breathe into that ease and softness. Notice the safety that is connected to that ease.

Now bring your awareness deeper into the body, letting it drop down into the chest. Connect with the crown of your heart—the top of your heart. Notice the space and comfort in this part of your body. Feel the strength and security on the top of your heart; let it be the harbor of safety in your chest. As you do this, let the safety and security you feel at the crown of the heart expand, taking up more space in your chest, creating a deeper sensation of ease, security, and bold tranquility.

As you stay connected to the breath, allow your consciousness to drop even deeper now into the body, down into your abdomen, letting your awareness rest in your diaphragm, the place where your belly meets your ribs. Here, too, connect to the breath and feel the power at the core and center of your body and being. Breathe into your power, letting it swell and take up a bit more space. Let yourself connect to the core of your body, breathing into the safety that comes with connecting to your own inner strength. Stay connected to this power and find ease and security in being in contact with it. Breathe. Stay here for a moment.

Finally, let your consciousness and breath drop deeper into your body, resting in the root of your pelvic floor. Feel the grounding force and inherent safety of being rooted low in the body. Connect to the spaciousness here and allow yourself to slow the breath a little more, letting it naturally drop deep into the body and fall out as it wishes. For a moment, visualize the root of your body connecting to the seat beneath you, moving down into the ground beneath you and into the earth below it. Breathe as you allow the sensation of safety to wash over you and through you. Feel the grounding of your root, the power of your core, and the spaciousness of your heart filling your body with strength and ease. As you do breathe into this, let that safety move and expand throughout your body. Let it enter into places or spaces that normally feel unsafe, tense, uneasy, or where you hold on to fear. Allow the safety you feel in the center of your being to expand out through your body, occupying more space, allowing the breath to move it into your arms, wrists, and hands. Let the safety move down your thighs, knees, calves, and feet, dropping all the way to your toes, and up to the very top of your head. Let the deep and unquestioned sense of safety emanate throughout the body, letting this feeling and sensation, wherever you feel it strongest, be imprinted in the mind and memory of your body as a place you can return to when needed. Let yourself rest easy for a moment in this sensation, enjoying the breath, enjoying the strength and suppleness. When you're ready, slowly return to your surroundings, remaining connected internally to the sensation and experience of safety in your body.

PART III

CHANGING YOUR RELATIONSHIP BEHAVIORS

8

CONFLICT

Your wounds store a tremendous amount of information. In the last several chapters we've worked hard to glean that valuable information from those wounds. Examining our past experiences for present-day insights is a painful yet powerful process. But here's the exciting part. Now you get to put all that knowledge into practice in your current and future relationships . . . and eventually shift to healthier, more satisfying behaviors.

There's no better place for us to be putting that hard-won wisdom about ourselves into practice than in examining conflict—the one constant in all our interpersonal associations and the point where so many of our best intentions about our behavior start to weaken.

We all engage in conflict, so why does it seem so fraught with peril? Well, for one thing, most of us did not grow up with healthy models of conflict. If you grew up experiencing control, conditional love, abuse, distraction, intolerance, and shame as a result of conflict, you probably didn't learn constructive ways to settle differences. Which means that when you're in conflict today, unhealthy behaviors often become your go-to way of engaging or responding. Perhaps you mimic what you saw or you try desperately to avoid conflict at all costs, creating a different set of issues you likely haven't considered.

Yet, and I know this will sound strange, conflict is also an attempt at *connection*. A lousy one, but an attempt, nonetheless. Think about why you start that same fight again and again. What are you hoping will happen? Do you want to feel more disconnected at the end of it? Are you anticipating that you will feel more sadness once it's done? Of course not. You hope that the other person will hear you at last, will finally understand what you've been trying to convey, will become aware of the pain that you've been sitting with, and will make the necessary changes.

And as peculiar as it might be, conflict can be a gateway to connection, intimacy, and our origin wound healing. The key is that we need to learn how to engage in conflict in a way that either acknowledges the wounds that have been activated or that avoids activating those wounds in the first place. We need to participate in *constructive conflict*.

Constructive conflict is when you engage others with the conscious goal of being seen, heard, or understood—and you offer the same to them. It's when you connect with your true emotional needs and clearly define the desired outcome on the other side of the conflict.

Think of it this way: creating conflict is often a way to try to bridge some kind of gap between you and the other person. Whether you bridge that gap or widen it depends on how consciously rather than unconsciously you engage in the conflict.

The conscious engagement of conflict is easier said than done. I practice this all the time, and yet sometimes I still throw all my tools out the window. I'm back to proving my point and doubling down. I share this with you because your goal isn't perfection. Your aim is to become a little more aware each time you find yourself in conflict. You will still be human and there will still be things that set you off. Having realistic expectations for yourself is important for your growth.

Let's take a closer look at how to achieve this kind of healing. It's possible.

I Want to Be Seen, Heard, and Understood

With the exception of those who are unable to feel empathy, almost every person I've ever met wants to feel seen, heard, and understood. But when that doesn't happen, it's easy for conflict to arise.

At the core of being understood is the feeling of being deeply known. If you have ever had the experience of feeling understood, it's probably because you felt the other person took a real interest in you and in what you had to say. This leaves most people feeling important, valued, prioritized, and safe. The person might have paid close attention, asked follow-up questions, shown no defensiveness or reactivity, and reflected back to you what they heard you say. It's a beautiful and profound experience when it happens. But if that scenario sounds foreign to you, you might think about all the times you haven't felt understood and consider what stands out to you there.

There are plenty of reasons you might not have felt understood growing up. Parents might have made hurtful assumptions about you, they might have shown little interest in your life, or they might have ignored you when you spoke. Maybe they were outright invalidating or told you that children were meant to be seen and not heard. They may have criticized the differences between you and them, instead of taking the time to get to know the real you and your dreams. Or they may have become defensive when you expressed yourself and turned your feelings around on you, blaming you for being difficult or ruining your time together.

My client Carly shared with me that her parents assumed that she was extroverted like her older siblings, and they would often pressure her to be more like her sisters. "They never listened to me when I told them that I was introverted and a highly sensitive person. I would tell them this repeatedly and it just fell on deaf ears."

Parents will occasionally miss the mark, of course. That's to be expected. They're never going to see, hear, and understand things perfectly. They won't always say the right thing or connect to everything that's being shared. But *how* they bring their concerns, differences, and wishes for you forward makes a huge difference. Your parents might not agree with something that you do, but you can still feel seen, heard, and understood. They might not support a decision that you're making, but they might understand why you're making it. Or they might not agree with your choice of lifestyle but still hear you out and accept your decision.

But sometimes parents *really* don't get it right. Sometimes parents prioritize themselves, which blocks them from seeing, hearing, or understanding their children. Parents have their own wounds and their own limitations that, when left unresolved, eventually just pass the pain on to us. If conflict is to have a chance at turning into connection, intimacy, and healing, then we must understand how our present relationship to conflict was built on the foundation of our wounds.

Simply put, our wounds have a lot to do with the way that we engage or create conflict.

How Conflict Begins

There are countless ways conflict gets initiated. When you consider all the instances of conflict that have ever made you upset or reactive, I imagine you could come up with many examples: from being criticized to having your concerns dismissed to being controlled or spoken down to.

Did you notice how the instances above focus on what the *other* person was doing? It's more palatable to read it that way first. But the reality is, conflict can be initiated either by you *or* by the other person. Conflict doesn't arise because everyone around you is doing not-so-great stuff. Sometimes conflict starts because *you* are the one who is engaging unhealthily. Oof indeed, but I know you're here for the hard work.

Regardless of whether you're engaging in conflict in response to someone else's reactivity or whether you're initiating the conflict on your own, what's leading the charge is your emotional reactivity, and if you're not paying close attention, this reactivity can quickly derail a conversation. It is often a result of a wound getting activated at the onset of conflict. As we'll see, if you tend to the wound *first* and acknowledge the emotional need behind it, you can begin to move away from knee-jerk reactivity and pivot toward being genuinely seen, heard, and understood.

But let's begin by looking at the ways conflict gets initiated to better understand the patterns of how our reactivity to being activated gets us off track. This work builds on the work of Dr. John Gottman's "The Four Horsemen of the Apocalypse" and his four markers of relational failure. You're probably going to recognize yourself in one of these five scenarios, so buckle up, be kind to yourself, and allow what will be revealed to be revealed.

STOP BEING SO CRITICAL

"I don't know if we're going to make it. This just isn't working." Veronica came into therapy one day frustrated and worried that her new partner was going to call it quits on a relationship.

"Listen, I ask for the simplest things and he makes a huge deal about it. I'm just over it. Yesterday I asked him to grab dinner on his way to my place, and then I called him back to ask him if he could quickly stop into a grocery store to pick up a few things that I would need for this morning. No big deal. Like four items, just so I could have my breakfast and coffee the way I like it."

Veronica's tasking of her partner was one of the ways that she tried to get him to prove that she was worthy. *If he will make another stop and pick up the groceries, it will show me that I am worthy, that I am important enough for him to do the things I ask him to.* This would make a deposit into the "I am worthy" bucket.

But the moment Veronica felt resistance, pushback, or boundaries being set was the moment her worthiness wound would open up. "He said he was tired from a long day at work and didn't have time to go to the grocery story after he picked up the takeout," she complained to me. "How selfish! What's it going to take him? Max twenty minutes in there?" She was getting heated again just recounting the story to me.

Veronica's partner couldn't understand what was beneath the request or why his refusal to make a second trip out after a long day at work was so crucial. He saw her request as insensitive and probably thought to himself, *Why are you asking me to do something else when you know I'm exhausted after a long day at work? You don't need these things tomorrow. You'll be fine.* He set a boundary, causing a chain reaction that would ultimately lead to the whole situation escalating. The result: Veronica's worthiness wound was instantly raw and activated, triggering her protection response: to become reactive and aggressive and cause a fight without giving any context.

This seemingly innocuous event—his boundary around a second stop to get the creamer for her morning coffee—caused a major blowout between Veronica and her boyfriend. Things escalated from there. Veronica began to hurl criticisms at her partner, not just about this event but about his character and who he was as a person. And as we all know, an attack on your character is no joke. It's cutting and damaging; this is where significant relational damage occurs in a conflict. No wonder so many people become defensive if they're being criticized constantly. It makes sense, doesn't it? The more you criticize the other person, the more the other person shuts you out, speaks up in self-defense, or criticizes you back.

In Veronica's case, she and her partner got stuck in a criticism-defense loop that only escalated things. She insulted his character and then he defended himself. Then they'd switch. This went on for hours and got them nowhere. Have you ever been there before? It's exhausting mentally, emotionally, and physically and leaves you feeling disconnected from your partner. And on the other side of it, it can leave you questioning everything.

I understood why Veronica was worried about the status of their relationship. She and her partner found themselves in this cycle often, and the conflict exhausted her. And unbeknownst to her, it had also left her worthiness wound raw. But here's the thing: we can't heal our wounds if we don't even know they're activated in the first place.

I slowed Veronica down and asked her if she could identify what wound had been activated before the conflict started. Veronica had identified her worthiness wound long before, so this language was familiar to her.

"I know it's worthiness, but what happened that made me question my worthiness to him?" she asked.

"Well, what did it feel like when he said no to you about the groceries?"

"Clearly I didn't like it. But what's your point?"

"Is your worth dependent on what others will do for you?" I asked. "Do you decide your worth based on how willing or unwilling another is? Do you base your worth on whether a person will stick around no matter how much you push them, test them, or try them?"

I was making my point. Veronica could see that when her partner said no, her worthiness wound heard: *No, because you're not worthy enough for me to do this for you.* Instead of vulnerably bringing that forward, she moved into attack mode. She bypassed seeing, hearing, and understanding herself. She moved straight into trying to get him to apologize, to admit he was wrong and she was right, and to ask her for forgiveness. This was her attempt at being seen, heard, and understood—but it was failing miserably.

Criticism doesn't move you toward what you want, it moves you away from it. Criticism doesn't encourage others to see, hear, and understand you. Instead, it encourages them to protect themselves more and move away from collaborating with you. Instead of conflict turning into connection, it was turning into disconnection.

When was the last time you were critical? Which wound got activated that moved you toward criticism? And what were you trying to communicate beneath the criticism?

When was the last time you felt criticized? Can you think about what wound got activated? And then how you reacted to that criticism? What were you trying to get across that perhaps you didn't communicate well?

STOP BEING SO DEFENSIVE

"I knew I shouldn't have gone home for the holiday."

I hadn't seen Ally since before Christmas, and this was our first session back to start the new year. Ally is the young woman whose mother had accused her of flirting with her father when she was a teenager.

For months Ally had been trying to decide whether she'd go to her parents' home for a few days to celebrate the holiday with them as a family. It had been a decade since the psychotic episode or any new accusations. Her mom had subsequently done her own therapy over many years, and she was a very different woman from the one Ally knew back then. Since Ally had been working on vulnerability, she was considering going home and sharing with her mom what that experience had been like for her growing up. She had never spoken to her mother about this before.

Ally knew this was a risk. We had prepared for the conversation, discussing expectations, fears, insecurities, and worst-case scenarios, but Ally felt ready.

"What happened?" I asked.

"I did everything we talked about, but she got defensive immediately. I didn't criticize her at all. I shared what my experience was growing up and told her how scary it was for me when she accused me of flirting. I even said that I understood where she was coming from and how sad her sexual trauma was. But she didn't want to hear it. She kept turning it back around on me, telling me that I didn't remember things correctly and saying that I had a great childhood and that she was an incredible mother who sacrificed so much and that she couldn't believe how ungrateful I was. I hung in there for a while. I kept trying to get her to hear how scary the experience was for me, but she just couldn't."

Defensiveness is the act of avoiding ownership, responsibility, and accountability. It usually includes making excuses, changing the focus, claiming innocence, or behaving in other ways that might allow you to skirt responsibility.

Seen through a compassionate lens, defensiveness is an attempt at protecting the self from criticism, and it might even be an attempt at changing the other person's mind about you. If that person's perspective is unflattering, you might sensibly respond: *I'm not bad. I'm not selfish. I'm not a monster.* But criticism met with defensiveness just throws you into a vicious cycle that can quickly erode the relationship.

I could see how upsetting her mom's defensive reaction to Ally's attempts to talk about her nonexistent childhood flirting was for Ally. As much as we had prepared for anything to happen, Ally was hurt and disappointed. She wanted her mom to acknowledge her pain. In her ideal world, she'd get an apology from her mom and some ownership and accountability. But what she got instead was defensiveness.

"How did you respond?" I asked.

"At first I got louder, just trying to talk over her. Obviously that doesn't work, but I couldn't help myself. I kept screaming at her to just listen to me, but eventually I gave up and shut down. Her defensiveness felt like an attack. I changed my flight for the next morning. I couldn't get out of there soon enough." Ally was bumping up against her mom's limitations. She tried different types of adaptation strategies, from being kind, thoughtful, and deliberate with her words to getting louder and trying to speak over her mom, but nothing worked. Nothing was going to get her to feel seen, heard, and understood. Eventually she would resign herself and leave.

Sometimes wounds get activated by the same people who put them there in the first place. Ally was trying to repair her relations with her mom. Part of her healing work was to become more vulnerable, and she really wanted her mom to understand the impact she'd had on Ally while she was growing up.

"If I can get her to understand this, it will feel so good."

Ally was attempting to bare her wound to her mom, hoping that her mom would be able to put her defensiveness aside and connect with her daughter's pain. But she couldn't. She needed to protect her own self more than she needed to connect with Ally. She needed to preserve her own image of herself as a mother more than she wanted to understand her daughter's pain.

"How could I have avoided the conflict? Should I just never go back to visit my parents ever again?" Ally asked.

There *are* times when being cut off from others makes sense, but more often, the work is in accepting that another person won't change. Sometimes the work is changing the way you relate to that person's inability to change. Sometimes the healing is in releasing the hope that they will see you, hear you, and understand you, and then in choosing how to engage in that relationship moving forward.

But before we found solutions, I wanted Ally to see how her safety wound got activated. Her mother's defensiveness turned into such an ordeal that it took the focus away from Ally's vulnerability, her need to feel safe, and her desire to have her mom connect with the pain from the past. Her mom's defensiveness activated Ally's wound. She tried to stick with her vulnerability, but eventually she started engaging with the conflict by yelling, then shutting down, and then getting out of there as quickly as she could.

"Why didn't I just breeze over it and stay the entire trip? I'm so dramatic. I didn't need to leave that way." Ally was revealing some embarrassment and shame.

"I think you left that way because you weren't feeling safe."

My response made sense to her. Tending to her safety wound, at least for now, meant choosing not to engage with her mom about her wounds. It meant leaving an environment that wasn't bearable for her. Ally chose to disengage from the conflict and to continue to tend to her wound and connect with her own grief, instead of asking her mother, who couldn't or wouldn't, to try to acknowledge her grief. Healing meant grieving the fantasy of the type of mother she had craved growing up, as well as the vision she had for her mother today. There was a lot of loss there for Ally, but in the loss was also her healing. What she was releasing offered her clarity and certainty. What she let go gave her a sense of peace.

When was the last time you were defensive? What wound had been activated when the defensiveness presented? And what were you trying to communicate through the defensiveness?

When was the last time you experienced someone being defensive with you? What wound got activated inside of you then? How did you react to their defensiveness? What were you trying to communicate that you perhaps didn't communicate well?

STOP BEING SO CONTROLLING

Isabel and Jo were ten minutes late to their session. They came running in and apologized.

"I'm so sorry we're late." Isabel said. "We lost track of time."

Isabel and Jo are the friends turned lovers who moved from Spain to New York City for graduate school. I learned that they were late to therapy because they had been caught up in a fight.

"Do you want to tell me about the fight you had?"

Jo launched right in. "I am not okay with being controlled. I know we keep talking about this, but it's getting to be too much. I can't just keep my life small so that I don't ever upset Isabel. I can't just make sure she's fine all the time so that she doesn't get triggered. *I'm* triggered. I don't want to come home within fifteen minutes of her texting me. I don't want to get off my phone just because she needs my attention."

Isabel and Jo were back at it. This conflict felt like the same old conflict yet again, just with some slightly different details. And when you get lost in the details, you better believe that you'll be right back another time, too. That's because, as Dr. Susan Johnson, creator of Emotionally Focused Therapy, puts it, "most fights are really *protests* over emotional disconnection." These strategies are unconscious attempts at dealing with the fear of losing connection. It's much nicer when you put it that way, but the reality of it is that you don't usually experience conflict this way when you're in it.

What had set off their conflict was Isabel telling Jo to put her phone away. "She said, 'You've been on it all day; don't you think it's time to take a break?' in the rudest tone ever. No, I don't. I think I'm a grown-ass woman who can choose how long she wants to be on her phone." Jo was not having it. "I am so over your prioritization wound. I have wounds, too, you know. You don't seem to ever consider that." She was directing this straight at Isabel.

If you remember, you learned a lot about Isabel's prioritization wound, but you didn't learn much about Jo. In our work together, Jo had shared how controlling her father was. He was very strict, setting down many rules for his daughter, and if they were not followed perfectly, she was punished. He was mean, would take away access to her phone and computer, and would ground her for months. This would happen if she missed her curfew by one minute. "Even when I had a legitimate excuse, it didn't matter. And then, when he found out I was gay, the control and punishment was on another level. He thought it was a choice, so he'd try to control me into choosing differently. But all it did was leave me feeling like I didn't belong."

Both Isabel and Jo had wounds activated in their fight: Isabel's prioritization wound and Jo's belonging wound.

"Why do you think things escalated between you and Isabel?" I asked.

"Because she's controlling." Jo replied.

"Well, maybe. I'm not sure. What you told me is that she pointed out that you were on your phone and asked if you thought it was time to take a break. I didn't hear the tone, so I'm missing a detail, I know. But it sounds like she was making an observation and then asking a question."

"It felt like control."

"Okay, and what's familiar about that?"

Jo knew that she was experiencing Isabel as her father. Isabel's prioritization wound and Jo's belonging wound went head-to-head. Isabel's need to feel prioritized was in question when Jo was on her phone, and Jo's need for freedom while still being in a relationship was in question when Isabel questioned her social media usage. *Can I have some space and still belong in this relationship? I don't want to accept being controlled in order to feel that I'm a part of something.*

Whew. Two wounds activated at once. Two people wanting to be seen, heard, and understood simultaneously. Two people going about it ineffectively. Two people finding themselves in a conflict loop and feeling more disconnected.

In that session we slowed things down a bit, but they were still too riled up to really see things clearly. It wasn't until the next session that we could really break it down.

I had each take a turn connecting to their wound and expressing that to the other person. They shared what felt familiar, and instead of each accusing the other of something, shifted the focus back to what their emotional needs were.

Isabel went first. "I honestly just want to spend time with you and for you to want to spend time with me. I love spending time with you, and I was missing that. I'm sorry I didn't know how to communicate that differently."

Jo went next. "I want freedom to just do the things I want to do sometimes. I love spending time with you, too, but I also love spending time with me and doing mindless things that help me disconnect from all the stuff we have going on. I want to know that I can do things for myself and still be a part of this relationship. Sometimes I feel like I'll only be accepted as a part of the relationship if I do what you want and need. That feels like control, and it's too stifling for me."

Can you see how the emotional needs brought each right back to their origin wounds? Isabel's emotional needs focus on wanting to be a priority. She wants to spend time with Jo, and she wants Jo to want to spend time with her. And Jo's emotional needs focus on belonging. *I want to know I can do things for myself and still be a part of this relationship.* I want to be me and still belong.

They had both done a beautiful job expressing themselves to each other, but just as important was the fact that they were acknowledging themselves, their wounds, and their needs well. This is where the pivot can happen. This is where change can take place. Tending to our wounds disrupts our reactivity, preventing us from lapsing into the same conflict cycles. It doesn't always happen in the moment when things are hot, but if we have a commitment to growth, there is the opportunity to circle back and see what it is that's being missed.

Conflict, when done well, can move people toward deeper connection, intimacy, and healing with themselves and each other. I see it as a flag in the sand that lets each of us know that something very important is going on beneath the surface. Conflict is one of the greatest indicators that on the other side of slowing down, curiosity, and openness is something unhealed that's crying for your attention.

When was the last time you were controlling? Can you think about what wound got activated for you that moved you into reactivity? What were you trying to communicate through the control, and why was control the vehicle you used?

When was the last time you felt controlled? Can you think about what wound got activated? How did you react to that control? What were you trying to communicate that you perhaps didn't communicate well?

STOP BEING SO CONTEMPTUOUS

"I'm quitting. Seriously. I'm out of there. I can't stand this job. I can't stand *him*." Carl was pissed. He was in for a midday session and had just come from work where his boss had done something to set him off.

Carl is the navy brat whose controlling father had him and his siblings do early morning military workouts.

"Do you need to do a conscious rant?" I asked. This is where you just let it rip. No need to be polite, no need to watch what you say— just vent and let it out. A rant can feel really relieving and release a lot of energy that's being stored. Carl was ready!

"Honestly, I've been fantasizing about the way I'll quit. What's the best way to put him in his place? What can I do to embarrass him or mortify him? He's such an asshole, and I'm so sick of him and his stupid face. He thinks he's all mightier than thou; he's barely older than me, a total idiot, and doesn't know how to manage people. He's so condescending, always being degrading and sarcastic toward me. I'm so ready to quit."

Carl took a breath.

"How'd that feel?" I asked.

"Yeah, a little better. Thanks."

"So what happened? What's been going on at work? It seems like something happened right before our session."

"It's been going on for a while. He puts me down in front of others, is really controlling, and needs to micromanage everything. Today he left me off an email that I've asked him to keep me on many times. It just set me off and I told him he's an asshole and then we got into it."

Contempt is criticism to the max. It's the most destructive way we engage in conflict, and for couples it's the greatest predictor of relational failure. When people are being contemptuous, they're being disrespectful, sarcastic, and condescending. They speak down to the other person and often take a one-up position, where they see themselves as better than and the other person as less than. Contempt can include abuse, as we talked about in chapter 7, and it's common for the person on the receiving end of contempt to feel worthless, disregarded, and despised.

The conflict between Carl and his boss had apparently gotten pretty heated, so much so that people had to pull them apart. No punches had been thrown, but they were up in each other's faces hurling insults. Carl was rightfully frustrated, but he also knew that his reaction was inappropriate. *There* was his neon sign. Of course no one wants to be spoken down to and controlled, but his reactivity was alarming.

"Carl, why do you think you reacted this way?"

"Is him being an asshole not the answer?" He snickered.

I smiled back but nudged him further. "What's familiar about what happened? Does the way your boss behave remind you of anything or anyone?"

It clicked in for him. His boss was reminiscent of his father. Carl felt controlled, spoken down to, and disregarded by him, and the way his boss went about things made Carl feel like he wasn't a part of the team. He was struggling to feel like he belonged.

It took a little time, but Carl was able to identify that his belonging wound had been activated by his boss's leaving him off the email, and he moved straight into conflict in an attempt to be seen, heard, and understood.

"Well, what am I supposed to do when he does these things?" Carl asked.

For starters, I wanted Carl to slow down and connect with his wound first. The way his boss was treating him and speaking to him was not okay. But what his boss was doing was offering an opportunity for Carl's wound to be revealed to him. It's an odd offering, I know, but it's still an offering.

"Witness the wound, Carl. Instead of engaging with him right away, go inward instead. Don't tend to the outside relationship, tend to the inner one. You're not going to get what you need from him in that moment, I can promise you that. I don't know if you'll ever get what you need from him, but it certainly won't happen this way. Can you try it? Take a moment to see, hear, and understand why you got upset."

"I feel disrespected and degraded. I feel like he puts me down and treats me differently from the others. I feel intentionally left out, and if I'm being honest, it makes me feel angry."

"That's good," I said. "When someone is treating you with contempt, it's important to set a clear and direct boundary with them. What you did was become emotionally reactive, and I get it. Honestly, what you're describing is enough to make most people become reactive. But your work is to connect to yourself and then engage your boss differently. You want to be seen, heard, and understood, right? So you need to become clear with yourself and then with him if you're going to have a chance at that."

"What if he still doesn't listen or care?" Carl had a fair point.

"He might not. There's no guarantee here, but what changes is the way you honor yourself and see yourself in this. What changes is that you become emotionally attentive instead of emotionally reactive. That's the victory. Whether your boss changes his ways or not is out of your control. Your work is to be responsible for you. You *may* choose to leave this job if things don't change, but we're not there yet. Right now all that I want you to think about is the boundary that you are setting with him and how you would bring that forward."

Carl gave it a shot. "I don't appreciate being spoken to the way you speak to me, and I don't appreciate being left out. It feels degrading and condescending. I want to be treated respectfully and I want to feel a part of this team. If there are things that I'm doing that you want me to change, please talk to me privately about that."

Carl's work is to engage the conflict differently. What he did was get caught in a conflict loop with his boss. They went back and forth, and it had gotten them nowhere. The work is moving away from emotional reactivity and moving toward emotional tending. It's the only way to end the cycle. Sometimes you can do emotional tending together, if it's an intimate relationship you care about, and sometimes you do emotional tending on your own, such as with Ally, who was working on seeing herself even if her mom couldn't. Tending to your own emotions helps establish safety, and it focuses you on being seen, heard, and understood even if you're the only one doing it.

When was the last time you were contemptuous? Can you think about what wound got activated for you that moved you into that space? What were you trying to communicate through the contempt?

When was the last time you felt contempt from another person? Can you think about what wound got activated when you experienced another person's contempt directed at you? How did you react to that contempt? What were you trying to communicate that you perhaps didn't communicate well?

STOP STONEWALLING

"I'm exhausted, and I don't want to be here, no offense." It was clear how shut down Mark was.

As discussed earlier, Mark and Troy had issues around trust. Troy got upset with Mark for not standing up for him at a party, but Mark himself had a worthiness wound stemming from receiving conditional love from his parents, and it had just been activated.

"This is what he always does," said Troy. "When the conversation becomes too much, he just shuts it down and won't engage. It's maddening. We were arguing last night and then he just got up and left the apartment. Didn't say anything to me. Just left. Turned off his phone and didn't come back for hours. I was asleep by the time he got back. It's outrageous."

Mark was engaging in stonewalling, a type of withdrawal that happens when people want to avoid conflict. They go to great lengths to put up a high stone wall, thus ensuring there is a lot of separation between them and the other person. This is done as a form of protection, but it is often triggering and destabilizing for the other person and can cause conflict between the two.

Troy couldn't get ahold of Mark. He didn't know where he was. He didn't know when he'd return. Troy was left in the dark, and although it's never great to be left in the dark, it's especially difficult when you're in the middle of a conversation that feels important to you.

"What were the two of you talking about?" I asked.

"Money. I was talking about how much we've been spending lately, and I feel like we need to be cutting back some. It wasn't even a fight. I just started the conversation, but then Mark shut it down. He didn't want to talk about it. I pushed a bit because we need to get on the same page, but he wouldn't respond. It irked me that he just kept looking down at his phone while I was trying to speak to him and then he got up and left."

Mark responded quickly. "I'm tired of having Troy point out everything I'm not doing up to his standards. I don't have his back well enough. I don't save money well enough. It's endless. I'm not interested in the conversation, so yeah, I left because it's the only way to make it stop."

Mark's worthiness wound was activated the moment Troy started to talk about something he thought Mark needed to do differently. It's so easy for a request or observation to go sideways. Even though Troy had explicitly said that *they* needed to cut back on the spending, Mark was hearing that *he* needed to. He was hearing that this was just another thing on a long list of things that he wasn't doing well. He was hearing that he isn't a good enough partner, which was activating his worthiness wound from childhood.

What Mark kept hearing from Troy was a pointing out of his lack of perfection, which meant that love, connection, and validation would be soon lost, too. Mark's learned way of protecting himself was by shutting down and disconnecting. It was a bit of a safe haven for him, but Mark's stonewalling would make things exponentially worse.

Both Mark and Troy were able to see how Mark's wound had gotten activated even though Troy was well intentioned in wanting to discuss the topic of money. Mark's emotional reactivity led him to stonewall instead of acknowledging the wound with himself and with Troy. This doesn't mean that Mark can't take a break from the conversation or do something soothing for himself, it just means that he acknowledges what's happening and communicates what he needs to do to regroup.

"If you had been aware of the wound activation, what might you have said instead?" I asked Mark.

"I guess I could have told Troy that I was feeling criticized. That it just seemed like it was another thing I wasn't doing well in his eyes and how that makes me feel unworthy of his love."

This was the start to emotional tending. When we exhibit vulnerability, emotions can be connected to, tended to, and met with still more vulnerability. When we articulate our emotional needs and connect to our wounds, as Mark did when he shared that he was feeling unworthy, the path forward opens up. This is similar to what Dr. Mona Fishbane calls the Vulnerability Cycle, and it helps us move from reactivity to reflectivity.

When was the last time you shut down entirely? Can you think about what wound got activated for you that moved you into that unhealthy coping strategy? What were you trying to communicate through the stonewalling?

When was the last time you were on the receiving side of stonewalling? Can you think about what wound got activated when that happened? How did you react to the shutdown? Even though there are plenty of times another person might stonewall you without being provoked, there are other times when it is provoked. Can you consider if you played any part in this? Were you doing anything to contribute? And what were you trying to communicate that you perhaps didn't communicate well?

Replacing Reactivity with Understanding

I remember once long ago hearing Dr. John Gottman say, "Behind every complaint there is a deep personal longing." We criticize and complain about our partners, our family members, even our friends when an emotional need of ours isn't being met. Instead of standing beside that emotional need, getting to know it, and bringing it forward, we move away from it, become reactive, and make it about the other person.

But our emotional needs often *are* our wounds. And when they are, it's especially important that we proceed with care. We thus need to recognize them and tend to them if we are to have any hope of exiting the conflict and reactivity loop. If we can identify and express our origin wound, we are well on our way to being seen, heard, and understood.

Think about a complaint or criticism you've uttered recently or one that you often offer. It doesn't matter about whom, but I want you to bring into focus something that you've been complaining about or critical of. It might sound something like: *They're so inconsiderate of my time. They're so controlling. They're always on their phone. They won't ever show me who they're texting. They spend all their money and don't save for our future.*

As you read the above complaints and criticisms, can you spot any wounds or hidden emotional needs? I read: *They're so inconsiderate of my time*—and hear a desire to be considered worthy. I read: *They're so controlling*—and see a belonging wound and a desire to be free to be as you are. I read: *They're always on their phone*—and see a desire to be prioritized. I read: *They won't ever show me who they're texting*—and see a trust wound. And I read: *They spend all their money and don't save for our future*—and see a safety wound. You get the point. Can you unpack your complaint to see if there's a wound there? Can you identify what your emotional need is?

Remember Veronica's big blowout with her partner? I asked Veronica if she could turn her complaints and criticisms of him into emotional needs, so that instead of being led by her wounds and reactivity, she would have the space and understanding to choose how to engage further. "This sounds dumb," she responded but smiled and went along with it. "Okay, but how?"

I walked her through the translation. Instead of *You're so selfish,* try *I want to feel important to you.* Instead of *You don't care about me,* try *I want to be considered.* Instead of *You're the worst boyfriend ever,* say *I want to feel like I matter to you.* "Are you getting the hang of it?" I asked. She nodded and proceeded.

Truth is, our complaints can be endless, but our emotional needs are pretty much always the same. They tie right back to our wounds. If you think about what you complain about and translate it into emotional needs, those needs will likely emphasize worthiness, belonging, prioritization, safety, or trust. They might emphasize wanting to feel seen, heard, and understood.

Now try the translation for yourself. Think about the last conflict or any recurring conflict that you have and consider the moments before the conflict started. Can you identify what wound got activated? And in what ways did you use or engage in conflict to try to be seen, heard, and understood? Did you become critical, defensive, contemptuous, controlling, or stonewall? Can you see what that was attempting to do for you? And how did that work out for you?

- The wound that got activated was _____.
- I can see that now because _____.
- I move into conflict because _____.
- But what that winds up doing is _____.

Okay, beautiful work. Now just a bit more.

- What I'm really feeling insecure about or questioning is _____.
- What I want the other person to really understand about me is _____.

- If I replace the criticism, defensiveness, contempt, control, or stonewalling with my emotional need, I learn that _____.

Remember, you're hurt. The thing that happened, whatever it was, is activating something familiar for you. That's raw, my friend. Can you connect to both the origin story and the reason this particular moment is so painful? Be gentle with yourself in this exploration.

Practice When You're Not in Conflict

As I tell all of my clients, trying to navigate conflict when you're in it is usually a losing proposition. I recommend exploring this when you're *not* in conflict, when there's some space between the conflict and your individual or joint curiosity around it. We're usually too worked up when we're in conflict to process it well. Our systems are responding to other things that feel like a much greater priority.

Imagine being activated and upset and then trying to ask yourself which wound is at play. Eye roll central. Imagine being super escalated and trying to translate a criticism into an emotional need. Fill in expletive here. If you're there, amazing, but if you're like most folks, laugh that off and give some separate time and space to work with your wounds so that your guidance and boundaries with them have practice outside of conflict.

And while you're getting curious, remember that others have wounds, too. It's just as important to know and acknowledge other people's origin wounds as it is to know and acknowledge your own. Of course, they are in charge of themselves, but in intimate relationships— whether with partners, family, or friends—one of the kindest things you can offer one another is to remember that they, too, have a rich history with an origin wound that might be flaring up right alongside yours. Even if they're not quite yet ready to face it.

When you use your daily practice to learn to navigate conflict better, you will find endless possibility and potential in connection and intimacy. What an incredible reframe to think that on the other side of conscious conflict is a deepening for both you and those you love.

9

COMMUNICATION

Your relationship can actually deepen and become more intimate through conflict when you replace reactivity with understanding. As you've already learned, reactivity keeps your wound raw and exposed, while understanding helps you begin to heal your wound. But if you want to turn conflict into connection, you will likely need to improve not just your fighting style but your communication style as well.

The truth is, you'll never be free from all emotional reactivity. Sometimes you'll initiate a conflict, and other times you'll respond reactively to others who initiate something. You can work on this and get better at handling it, but you're likely not going to arrive at some place in the future where absolutely nothing revs your engine. Make some space for the human experience. Remember that your reactivity and theirs provide really important information for both of you—once you start to notice it and communicate it to each other.

Dr. Alexandra Solomon says that one of the most important aspects of healthy intimate communication is relational self-awareness. She describes this as "the ability and willingness to look honestly at what tends to set you off in your intimate relationship and how you handle yourself when you feel upset." If you're like most of us, you've probably engaged more in linear thinking, which internally might sound something like: *You're so insensitive, I'm so unreliable, you never do what I ask you to do, this wouldn't have happened if you just cared more, this only happened because I'm such an idiot.* This narrow-minded type of thinking assigns blame or shame. It loses sight of the rich and complex stories each of us has. And yet when we're activated, it's so easy to go straight there. Absolutely zero connection happens when you're stuck in linear thinking.

On the other hand, systemic thinking takes into account our family origins and the past relationships that we've had, reminding us that there's a complex and rich story present in every moment. It offers us this perspective about others as well. What a gift to be able to see ourselves and others through that lens. What a gift to understand that what's happening right now is not just about *this* moment; it's about every moment that predates it. Can you imagine how much would change in communication if you could remember that about yourself and the other person? Can you imagine the depth of compassion, empathy, or grace that could exist?

So if your partner criticizes you, you hear not just a critique about something that needs to happen at home, but also all the criticism you've experienced before—from your parents, former partners, and beyond. The reaction you might have makes much more sense through a systemic lens than a linear one. And if your partner is aware of this, they might be able to navigate this differently with you, finding a moment of connection in what could have been a devastating rupture.

As I said at the beginning of this book, thinking about our origin stories and seeing the complexity of these family systems is not meant to offer an excuse. It doesn't make things okay when they're not. But having context *does* offer something. When we start to communicate from this position, we move away from the details or the need to be victorious in arguments, and we move toward a deep knowing that we are both hurting and we'd both like to be seen, heard, and understood. This improves the quality of our communication.

To Communicate or Not to Communicate

When a wound gets activated, you have two choices: communicate or don't communicate. When you don't communicate, your wound story has no chance of being acknowledged by another. But I would like to offer a caveat on the choice to communicate at all.

There are understandable reasons why you might avoid communication. Of course, the goal is to *communicate well,* but you also need to discern *with whom* you ought to communicate. Let me clarify right here and now that sometimes choosing not to communicate is the healthiest choice. Choosing not to communicate is not passive. It's an active decision that recognizes that even if you speak with kindness, consideration, and clarity, a conversation with a specific individual still might not be safe or healing for you. You might choose not to communicate if you know that it will cause you harm, as in the case of someone in an abusive relationship. You might choose not to communicate if the other person is going to engage in any form of manipulation or turn it back at you. And you might choose not to communicate if you've learned through experience that the other person is committed to not hearing you or is committed to defending their position. To choose not to communicate means that you won't be acknowledged by another, but it also means that you won't be hurt or harmed further. Sometimes that's the healing. Healing requires discernment. And sometimes the best choice is to honor yourself, move along, and find others who can hear you.

There's another reason to carefully consider the choice to communicate. You already know that you received an education about communication from your family and your past relationships. In a healthy family, communication is often clear, kind, considerate, calm, curious, grounded, honest, and direct. But *your* education might have been different from that, it might have been destructive rather than healthy. And if you do choose to engage in communication but your origin wound hasn't been identified yet, there's a much greater chance that you will use one of the many destructive styles of communication I describe below to deliver your linear perspective of blame or shame.

As we discussed in chapter 8, using a destructive style of communication will only reopen the wound and create a conflict loop. You'll still struggle to feel heard and understood. Better to back up and identify your wound first before communicating.

If you want to move toward healthier communication, the most obvious thing that needs to shift is that you need to get clear about what it is you *actually* want to communicate. This might seem like a no-brainer, but if you've ever wondered to yourself while you were in the middle of an argument what you were even fighting about or thought back to that fight from a few days ago and asked your partner *What were we upset about again?*, then you know how easy it is to be talking about topics far removed from what you ought to be talking about. I mean this lovingly, but before you say anything, before you even open your mouth, your job is to connect with what your message actually is.

Unblocking Communication

Of course, healthier communication is the goal, but before you reach that goal, you'll want to understand what keeps you from it. What blocks you from that clear, kind, calm, curious, grounded, and direct communication? And then ultimately, how can you move closer to it? Let's take a look at how passive, aggressive, passive-aggressive, and disorganized styles of communication can block you from being seen, heard, and understood, and how you can become the kind of communicator that others want to engage with and that you want to be.

HONOR YOUR VOICE

After an awful holiday with her family, Ally had kicked off the new year with meeting someone she was finally interested in. She had been dating for years but had never found a good match. This guy was different. Ally had been going with him for a few months and things were starting to heat up.

"Is it crazy that I think I'm falling in love with him?" she asked in one of our sessions. She was worried about the speed with which her feelings had developed, given that it had been only a couple of months and they had not had any conversations about exclusivity and had not created any agreements about their relationship.

"I feel like I need to slow things down. I don't want to get hurt. What if he's not interested in being exclusive or isn't feeling what I'm feeling?" she asked.

"Well, have you told him how you're feeling? Or have you talked about what you'd like to see happen in the relationship?"

"No, definitely not. Don't you think it's too early to do that?"

"I don't," I said. "I think clarity and direction are important. You're making a lot of assumptions about what he may or may not want or feel, but you've never even asked him where he's at. Maybe he's feeling the same way about you. Maybe he isn't. But either way there's some important information you're skipping over by avoiding a conversation that could clarify a lot for you."

Ally gave me a look that suggested that she saw my mouth moving and heard my words, but that she'd pass on my proposal. "I just don't want to be *that* girl. I feel like I need to just let it do its thing."

"Okay, so let it do its thing and see how it feels," I responded.

Ally was shocked. I could see the "wait, you're letting me off the hook" expression on her face. But I wasn't letting Ally off the hook; she just wasn't ready yet. She needed to experience more.

A week later Ally showed up for her session. "It's eating me alive.

I saw him twice since last week and I'm so into him. What do I do?!? I want to be exclusive with him. Ugh, this is torture!"

Ally was a passive communicator. She avoided hard conversations at all costs. She would rather keep it in than let it out. Most passive communicators avoid expressing themselves and sharing how they *really* feel. They try not to disagree with others because they are afraid that conflict will arise or the conversation will go in a direction they don't want it to. The idea of sharing how she felt and then having to possibly face the disappointment that he wasn't feeling the same way was too much for her to handle.

"I just can't. It's not worth it. I just need to be fine with it being unclear."

Ally, like many passive communicators, had convinced herself that sharing how she felt just wasn't worth it. She was prioritizing his experience, deferring to what she *thought* he would want, and trying to present herself as go-with-the-flow flexible even though she was feeling far from it. *This* was happening at the expense of her.

"Ally, what are you afraid will happen if you say something?" I asked.

"I don't know. Maybe he'll get upset or end it. Maybe he'll think I'm just ruining a good thing by trying to put a title on it."

Ally's safety wound was being revealed. So many folks with safety wounds become passive communicators. Their past experiences have taught them that it's not safe to share, speak up, or ask for things. They learn that when they do speak up, they'll often be met with hostility, defensiveness, attempts at domination, abuse, criticism, or contempt. To avoid *is* the safety. To share lacks the safety.

"When has speaking up been unsafe to you before?" I asked.

"With my mom?" she asked.

"I think so, Ally. What have you learned about communication from your mom?"

"That it's not safe," she replied. "That I won't be heard, that it will turn into something worse, that I should have just left it alone and not said anything."

"That's right," I said. "You learned that communicating with your mom isn't safe. And that's true. We saw that again just a few months ago over the holidays. With your mom there isn't space for you to share openly and trust that it will be received well. But avoiding communication with everyone isn't the answer, either. You have to learn how to discern with whom you share and then muster up the courage to communicate what it is you really want to say."

Ally was ready now. She still didn't love the idea, but she was beginning to see that moving toward clear and assertive communication was an important step in the right direction. Ally needed to acknowledge her safety wound, see how it was a constraint to her communication, and recognize that her passivity was not only blocking others from hearing, seeing, and understanding her, it was keeping her from fully witnessing and acknowledging herself. This work was a part of reclaiming her voice, which had been taken from her long ago in a family environment that wasn't safe for her.

"All right, just play along with me, okay?" I said. "Suppose you had perfect circumstances, meaning there's nothing to be afraid of and this conversation is going to go exactly the way you want it to, what would you want to communicate? Say it as if you're saying it to him."

"That I really like you and I'm not interested in dating other people. I guess I'm curious whether you feel the same way." Ally looked at me to see if I thought that sounded good.

"Great!" I said. "You shared how you're feeling, and you asked him a question about how he's feeling. More will be revealed based on how he responds, but this is a great start."

"But what if it's not perfect circumstances?" she asked.

"It's always perfect circumstances to honor your voice, Ally."

What Ally was caught in was a game of *I'll do it if . . .* This game is played by billions around the world every day. *I'll do it if* [*I get the outcome I want*]. There is so much power when we shift from *I'll do it if* to *I honor my voice no matter what.* Oof central.

Honoring your voice is not dependent on whether another person hears you or not. To honor your voice requires *you* to hear yourself—always. For Ally, this meant listening to herself and hearing that she wanted exclusivity. Honoring her voice meant sharing that with the guy she had been dating. It didn't matter whether he agreed or wanted that as well (although that was clearly a preferred outcome), what mattered was that she listened to herself and chose to bring forward what she wanted to say.

Strengthening your voice involves continual practice. When you've learned to avoid communication and take a more passive route, you've also learned to devalue your experience and your truth. As you step toward healthier communication, it's valuable to walk yourself through the same steps I walked Ally through:

What are you really trying to say? Don't beat around the bush. Don't apologize unnecessarily or take ownership for something you don't have to own. Become clear about your message. Most therapists support the use of "I" statements. These statements are about the self, as opposed to telling other people about themselves. Ally needed to shift from "I don't know if you want to be exclusive" to "I am feeling great about this relationship, and I would like to be exclusive."

Can you try it? What's something that you've been avoiding saying that you'd like to honor? Remember, I'm not asking you to speak this out loud to anyone right now. This is strictly about your honoring your voice to yourself.

- Something I've been avoiding saying is _____.
- What I want is _____.
- Acknowledging this for myself feels _____.

Next is understanding the constraint. The constraint is what keeps you from bringing it forward, from using assertive communication. For Ally, it's her safety wound. She doesn't know that it's okay to express and share herself. When she looks at her history, she sees a lot of evidence that supports the fact that when she does share, things go south. What's at play for you? What are you afraid will happen? Can you acknowledge how your history plays a role here?

- In the past, when I've voiced important things, what happens is _____.
- What that's taught me about sharing is _____.
- What I'm afraid will happen today is _____.

This next step is very important. This is the discernment step we've touched on. This is where you choose whether the environment and person are actually safe or not. This can be challenging and confusing, and if you're unsure, choose your own safety every time. This means don't bring it forward until you feel that it's safe. Because I'm not in the therapy room with you and don't know your story, I can't walk through discernment with you as fully as I'd like to, but for now, one thing that you can explore is noticing the difference in your body between feeling safe and *not* feeling safe. Can you imagine the comfiest, coziest, most free space or place you've ever been? This might be wrapped in a soft blanket in your bed. This might be on a hike you took during your favorite vacation surrounded by nature. Maybe it's when you're cuddling your dog. Or it might be when you're chatting with your dearest friend on the sofa.

- When I envision _____, I feel _____ in my body. Notice and note the sensations in your body.

Now envision something that scares you. Is it heights? Or maybe a tarantula crawling on you. Maybe it's that time you had to speak before a crowd or maybe it's the fear of enclosed spaces. Don't hang out here for too long, but I want you to notice the difference in the sensation.

- When I envision _____, I feel _____ in my body.

I am not suggesting that you don't lean into something just because you feel tension in your chest or your palms are sweating. Some of our greatest wins come when we face the hard conversations that make us nervous or do the thing we thought we'd never be able to do. But a good starting place is noticing what our bodies are telling us. Wisdom and healing come when we can figure out what to override and what not to, but for now it's important to just notice the difference.

For Ally, we looked at what we knew about the guy she had been dating. Even though her heart would race in session when we talked about sharing with him, all the evidence that she had of him said that he'd be able to hear her and respond to her without this turning into a fight. It didn't mean that she would get the response she was hoping for, but we felt confident that he'd stay kind, calm, and grounded.

Ally leaned into the conversation. She came back to our next session giddy. "He wants to be exclusive!" she exclaimed.

We both smiled. With time, Ally and her new partner would learn quite a bit more about each other. That's the beauty of communication and where it can lead you. It wasn't the right time yet for her to share with him why she leans toward passivity, but eventually she would start to share more of the details. Ally's commitment to healthier communication was a continual practice. She would lean toward passivity for a long time. You might find that to be true for you as well, but through repetition you might also learn that there *are* people who can, will, and want to hear your voice, and that it's safe to share it with them.

HONOR OTHERS

Trish came into the office and was ready to get into it. "I keep getting this feedback from friends, and I feel like I need to talk about it with you." Trish has cerebral palsy, and she grew up with parents who denied that there was something physically different about her when she was a kid.

"What's going on?" I asked.

"This isn't the first time I'm hearing this, so I need to pay attention to it. My friends think that I'm abrasive when I communicate. I'm too direct. I don't know, they say that I lack any sympathy or empathy when they ask me for my opinion." Trish paused. "Why ask for my opinion if you don't want it? Anyway, I want to look at this because obviously there's something there."

Trish was getting feedback about the way she was communicating. Her friends, people who loved her, were telling her that she wasn't demonstrating consideration, compassion, concern, and empathy when they spoke. They'd come to her to talk about their personal lives, their ideas about work, or their choice of an outfit for an upcoming date. And no matter what the topic was, Trish was insensitive and brash.

"They're calling me a harsh truth teller. Do you think that's true?" she asked.

"I'm not sure, Trish. Should we dig a bit?" I responded.

Trish gave me the go-ahead. "You know where I want to start us, right?" I asked.

"I'm sure it has something to do with my family." Trish chuckled.

I smiled back. "Well, can we look at communication in your family system?" I asked. "What did you learn about communication growing up?"

"That it was nonexistent," she replied. "It didn't happen. People avoided things and never actually acknowledged what I needed them to."

"And how did you feel about that?" I asked.

"I hated it. I resented it. I wanted them to just be direct with me. I wanted them to just call my cerebral palsy what it was. I wanted them to stop hiding behind things and stop trying to protect me from it. Their avoidance did so much more damage than their attempt at protecting me from something I already knew and felt."

Trish had taken a path of opposition when it came to communication. She had seen how her parents communicated with her and decided to do a one-eighty. *I'll never not be direct. I'll never avoid hard conversations. I'll always tell people how it is. I know how painful it is to have things withheld.* These were her silent proclamations. But what Trish didn't realize was that she had overcorrected. She had become an aggressive communicator.

There's no one way that a person with a belonging wound communicates, but what we know is that how you communicate will either be an attempt at belonging or an attempt at maintaining the narrative that you don't belong. Either you'll adjust yourself to try to fit in or you'll behave in ways that prove the story about your wound to be true.

Trish was communicating in a way that would ultimately prove her wound story true. Her pendulum swing was turning others off. What she saw as direct, others saw as aggressive. Friends started to leave her out of things and create some distance. This path of opposition was leaving Trish feeling like an outsider. Her wound was fully exposed, but this time she would have a say in how to tend to it.

"I know you want to be direct with people in your life, but I wonder if there's a middle ground. Do you think you can be honest and forthcoming while also considering the other person's experience?" I asked.

"Part of what was so hurtful for you growing up was the lack of consideration of *your* experience. You wanted your parents to connect to what *you* needed instead of what *they* needed. Do you think that in some ways you're repeating that? Your friends are asking for more sensitivity from you. Maybe part of your growth here is to honor what the other person needs, in the same way that you craved that long ago."

Trish sat with this. It resonated with her. "This is a lot," she said. "But I hear you and I know what you're saying is right."

Trish shared with me that she told a friend who was going through a breakup that the friend was an idiot for staying this long anyway and that it was best that the ex broke up with her, since she would never have left. Gulp. "Well, how would you have said it?" she asked me. Truth is, it could have been put a number of different ways, but what I offered to Trish was something like "I'm so sorry you're in pain. Breakups are hard, and I'm here if you want to talk about it." This could have done the trick.

What Trish had to come to terms with was that not being aggressive didn't mean being avoidant.

"There's a repair that needs to happen here, don't you think?" I asked. "These are dear friends of yours. People who have been in your life for a long time. People you trust and know love you. The fact that they can even offer you this feedback says a lot. What do you think you need to take ownership for and acknowledge?"

"I see how abrasive I've been. I need to acknowledge that I've been harsh and insensitive. It's been unfair to them, and I get why they'd want some space between us."

"Do you think it would be appropriate for you to give some insight as to why you've communicated so directly and abrasively in the past? In sharing how this has activated your belonging wound?"

Trish started to cry. In many ways, her friends had been her family. She was seeing that there was an opportunity to be vulnerable and tend to her wound *and* honor others.

Trish needed to replace her harsh and abrasive communication with concern, care, and empathy, but before she just waved some magic wand, she needed to understand what was blocking her from that gentler style. She repeated out loud, "Not being aggressive does not mean that I'm being avoidant." She would need to remind herself of this, but there was a truth in this statement that she was making room for. If she continued to see aggression as the antithesis of avoidance, she'd hurt others and herself. She needed to think about the other person's experience of her, instead of bulldozing her way in.

Isn't it incredible how our wounds can get activated at different points in our lives, but that in that activation there is an opportunity for us to move toward healing? Trish took a chance on expressing her vulnerability, and as we expected, her friends opened themselves back up to her.

The path forward for Trish might not be your exact path forward, but can you think about the ways in which your wound, whatever it is, affects the way you communicate with the people in your life? Consider the ways your desire to belong, like Trish's, affects the way you communicate. Do you go along with what everyone else wants so that you never rock the boat, making it easier for you to fit in? Are you more assertive, making sure you have a place at the table? Notice what you can. But might you also explore the ways that communication was modeled for you, how the adults in your life communicated with each other and you, and how that style of communication affected your relationship to belonging?

CONNECT TO YOURSELF AND OTHERS

Veronica was on time for her session. "How'd it go?" I asked. I was curious about whether she and her partner had been able to move through their conflict from the week earlier and whether she had tried expressing her emotional needs instead of the criticism she was voicing in session.

"I haven't spoken to him in a week," she responded.

"Oh? Why's that?" I asked.

"He knows I'm angry. He's tried reaching out to me, but I haven't picked up yet or responded to his texts. I'll probably answer in the next couple of days."

Veronica was being passive-aggressive in her communication. She was giving her partner the silent treatment and was making her statement that way instead of using her words. She was creating a hierarchy within her relationship, one where she was on top and her partner was beneath her, asking for forgiveness and apologizing for something that he didn't need to apologize for. This game was an attempt at keeping Veronica in control.

Passive-aggressive communicators indirectly communicate their feelings instead of openly expressing themselves. They might use words to say one thing but then use their behavior to communicate something else. One example is a person who says she's fine with something but then won't look at you when you speak to her. Or someone like Veronica, who shuts down access to herself entirely and won't use her words to communicate her anger or frustration toward you. Passive-aggressive communication withholds love and access to the person as a form of punishment.

"Why are you punishing him?" I asked.

Veronica didn't have an answer. We sat there for what I assume felt like eternity for her. I wasn't going to fill the silence between us. I wanted her to sit with that question and answer when she was ready.

"I guess I want him to hurt when I'm hurting." she said.

"You mentioned that you were probably going to respond to him within the next couple of days. How do you know when it's the right time to respond when you're punishing in this way?" I asked.

"I respond once he's pleading with me. It's when I know that he'll do anything to make it better. He'll do anything to make me forgive him and get back in my good graces."

Veronica's worthiness wound was obvious, but she couldn't see it yet. She used passive-aggressive communication to get the other person to a point where, desperate for connection, he would bend over backward for her, placing her on a pedestal. This in her mind made her feel worthy.

This is definitely NOT how you prove you are worthy. It's a way of asserting power over the other person. This creates the illusion of worthiness but simultaneously diminishes a relationship and the people in it.

But Veronica had learned that passive-aggressive communication got her what she wanted, or so she thought. When she behaved this way, she would get the upper hand. When people would fight to get back on her good side, she would then feel like she was good enough for them. She'd feel special and important, and she'd feel valued by the other person. Her passive-aggressive communication was designed to protect her worthiness wound, but what it did instead was eventually cause the end of relationships.

When Veronica's partner didn't pick up the groceries, her worthiness wound got activated. Her go-to reaction was to then become passive-aggressive: *I'm going to teach you a lesson and make it so uncomfortable for you that you will then prove to me how worthy I actually am.* But what happens in that situation is that Veronica never really has to feel her feelings and she never has to communicate about them. She never connects to herself or addresses her wound, and thus she has no way of truly connecting to her partner, of communicating her hurt, her feelings of unworthiness, to others. Without that connection to herself and her partner, she has no direction for healing.

Since this was her last shot at therapy, it was now or never.

"Your passive-aggressive communication is one of the things that's keeping you from feeling worthy," I said.

Veronica looked at me, shocked.

"How do you feel about yourself when you behave this way? How do you feel about yourself when you treat someone you say you care about this way?" I asked.

"I feel awful. I am disgusted with myself."

We sat there for a moment as I let her feel the impact of her words.

"What do you think feeling disgusted with yourself does to your worthiness wound?"

"It makes it worse," she answered. "I don't actually feel worthy of love and partnership when I behave this way. I actually think he should leave me."

Power and control are attempts at protection. But your wounds are not actually protected when you manipulate your way to power and control. Veronica didn't become more worthy because she forced people into behaviors that made her feel like she was. She'd feel more worthy if she could like who she was and stop engaging in behavior that made her ashamed of herself.

"I don't want to do this anymore," she said. "I do see how much I test people and how much I push them away. Even though in my heart of hearts I really want to believe I'm worthy, I can see how I'm really committed to proving that I'm not. The evidence I think I get is all just bullshit."

This was a big breakthrough for Veronica. It was painful and emotional. Her relationship did end, but in many ways, this was an important consequence for her to experience. She was committed to changing the way she spoke to people. When she was hurt, she would slow down and connect to what she really wanted to express. This required some processing before she spoke, but she'd look for her worthiness wound in her pain and notice her desire to quickly go to passive-aggressive communication. Instead of operating from a position of *How do I protect myself?* she shifted to *How do I connect to and protect this relationship?* Take that in.

Whatever the relationship is, what a beautiful question to consider. How do I want to speak to you and thus to protect *us*? Oof. Don't blow by this. There is me and there is you, and how we both feel and experience this moment is important. I know this can't happen in every moment of communication or conflict. When things get heated, it's hard, but if you even think about that question every once in a while, consider how much could shift in your relationship communication. And if you can think about that question before you state how you're feeling, what can that open up? To consider the *we* does not take away from your experience. This does not ask you to put others before yourself. It asks you to put your relationship right next to yourself.

Whatever wound you identify with, can you look at the ways your passive-aggressive communication style either tries to support the wound story or tries to deny it? Do you become passive-aggressive in an attempt to get others to read through the lines so that you don't have to confront something uncomfortable for you? And might you consider how the way communication was modeled for you in your family of origin impacts how you choose to engage with others today?

Remember, you can be on the same team. In fact, when you're not against each other, when it's not you versus me or me versus you, connection can replace disconnection. When we shift away from destructive communication, we give ourselves and others the opportunity to be seen, heard, and understood. We give ourselves and others the opportunity to see what's happening through that systemic lens again. This is a beautiful shift toward connection.

GET GROUNDED

Earlier in the book I discussed Miyako and Jin. Jin had a safety wound. While you don't have much backstory on Miyako yet, she has a prioritization wound. That might not be surprising to you, given their dynamic and her desire to have Jin prioritize an engagement and marriage.

"Some days Miyako is so level-headed and other days she's so in my face about our future. I thought we had agreed to take this step by step together." Jin was upset about the conversations they had been having outside of therapy and some of the conflicts they had found themselves in.

"Miyako, do you know what Jin is talking about?" I asked.

"Yes, he's upset that I'm making sure that we follow through on the conversations we agreed to have."

Jin jumped in. "That's absolutely not true. I'm not upset about talking about our path forward, I'm upset about the way you're talking to me. I'm upset that some days you seem so clearheaded and then other days you're in my face yelling at me, telling me that I need to get over my safety wound, mocking it, and other days you ignore me. This is not okay."

Miyako was engaging in a disorganized communication style. In the past, she had communicated one thing one day and another thing the next. But now she was going in and out of communication styles, communicating with care and concern one day, becoming aggressive another, and then being passive-aggressive the next. This did not make Jin feel safe, but I wanted to understand more about what was going on for Miyako.

Miyako grew up as the only child of two parents who were both preoccupied. Her parents were hard workers, but they put a lot of their time and energy into their work and didn't have much time for Miyako. Her father was also a big gambler, and any time away from work was spent with his addiction.

When he won money, he was kind, loving, and affectionate. He'd buy something nice for Miyako and would be in great spirits. He would want to talk about his day and was curious about the things going on in Miyako's life. But when he lost money, he was angry and unapproachable. He'd tell her to leave him alone and not bother him, often getting very angry about her desire for connection with him. She'd run to her mom for comfort, but her mom was too busy to care for Miyako's emotional needs.

I knew this about her childhood, so I had a feeling that Miyako's disorganized way of communicating was a repetition of what she grew up around. Miyako had been left with a prioritization wound, and she was using every style of communication in the book to force her way to prioritization.

Although there isn't one specific way that someone with a prioritization wound communicates, it makes sense that a person who wants to be prioritized might try anything to see what gets them the outcome they want. *If I'm avoidant, can I be prioritized then? If I'm aggressive, will that work? How about when I'm calm, cool, and collected? Still no?* Wash. Rinse. Repeat.

Miyako had tried it all with Jin. And although they were making some progress, it wasn't at a pace that felt good for her. Even though we were hard at work on their goals, Miyako's prioritization wound was activated, and in her attempts at communication, she was in effect throwing anything up against the wall to see what would stick. Not only was this method not working, it was also activating Jin's safety wound. Miyako's disorganized attempts to communicate with him were just driving him further and further into himself as he tried to find safety from what he experienced as chaos and threats, an experience he knew all too well.

Sometimes in therapy when you get to the root of something, it actually slows a process down. We start unearthing something that's been hidden for a long time, and an individual or couple who comes in to address a problem they think they can get an answer to within a few weeks finds it winds up taking longer. Unquestionably this can be frustrating, but it's much better to make a decision based on seeing the whole picture instead of just part of it.

"The pace we're going is really delaying the plan you had, isn't it?" I directed my question at Miyako.

She nodded.

I understood Miyako's frustration and also reminded her of why we had chosen to intentionally slow things down. "Miyako, what are you actually trying to communicate to Jin?" I asked.

She sat there for a few seconds and then looked up at me. "I don't actually know." She looked perplexed.

"Okay," I said. "What do you want Jin to communicate to you?"

"That I'm a priority to him. That this relationship matters to him." She knew the answer to that right away. "But he's not showing me that."

"Is he not showing you that or is he not showing you that fast enough?" I asked.

I could see that she didn't love the question, but she made some space for it. "I guess that it's not fast enough."

I asked this question because I had been working with Jin and Miyako for a while and I knew that Jin *was* prioritizing Miyako and the relationship. He was working tirelessly at moving toward engagement and doing it in an authentic way. He didn't want to just propose and get it over with. He wanted to propose because it came from a place of deep love, desire, respect, and mutual commitment for each other. He was so close, but Miyako's prioritization wound was getting activated in moments when she'd see other friends of hers getting engaged or married. She'd try to push Jin to propose by speaking to him calmly and with care at first. But Jin could feel that this wasn't authentic. She'd then become aggressive, and when that didn't work, she'd become passive-aggressive.

I noted with her that her disorganized style of communication was like her father's. "Have you ever noticed that before?" I asked.

Miyako's chin dropped slightly and she began to cry. "Oh, my goodness." She paused to try to collect herself, but the tears kept coming. Eventually she turned directly to Jin. "I'm so sorry. I know what that's like and I never want you to go through that. I guess that when I feel scared and unsure, I try everything I can to get your attention to prioritize me."

"But I am prioritizing you, Miyako. I love you. I am excited for our future together. I just want to get there in a way that is stable and sound for both of us."

Jin was being heartfelt. Miyako *was* scared. She didn't want to be a fool, and she didn't want to be embarrassed and disappointed at the end of this. But instead of bringing her fears forward so that they could both express themselves openly, she was communicating them in ways that created chaos, disconnection, and more doubt. This was something that she knew all too well from her childhood.

We held both of their wounds in that session, with one eye on Jin's safety wound and one eye on Miyako's prioritization wound. Both had to get clear on what they needed from each other in their conversations, and they both needed to communicate with each other in a grounded and clear way. Because they were both aware of their own and the other's origin wounds, they were starting to notice reactivity within themselves and each other and replace it with curiosity. This was impressive to watch.

Their curiosity opened up so many new conversations for them. They were committed to communicating with each other in honest, vulnerable, and transparent ways. Of course they had their moments of conflict and disconnection, but what they had built was strong and they both felt confident moving forward. Their yeses to each other were yeses they could actually trust. *That* was the victory. Anyone can say yes, but to feel a deep sense of confidence connected to the yes makes a huge difference. One that left Jin feeling safe and Miyako feeling like a priority.

Can you consider how to be grounded in your communication? And what it is that's blocked it in the past? Can you focus in on what you want to say rather than leading with disorganization or chaos?

Remember, the first thing you need to get clear on is what you're actually trying to say. What are you trying to communicate to the other person? This was something that Miyako had initially struggled with. If this is hard for you to identify, my next question to her might support in unlocking something for you, too. What are you hoping the other person communicates to you? That might get you a bit closer to your emotional need.

If you could replace a disorganized style of communication with grounded vulnerability and clarity while being, kind, honest, and direct, what's the sentence you'd like to share with them and what would you like to hear in return?

The goal is to be in relationships where we are honoring ourselves and the other people through grounded communication. To be able to bring our voice forward, even when it shakes, is a major victory. And to be able to do that while you simultaneously consider and care about the impact of the words on the other person is a beautiful expression of respect and love.

Getting Clear on What You Want to Say: The Path Forward

As you might have already guessed, any wound can match with any communication style. Someone with a safety wound, like Ally, might communicate passively in order to avoid conflict, but other people with a safety wound might become aggressive because it's the only way they believe they can keep themselves safe. They might think something like: *If I get bigger, louder, and more aggressive than my enemy, then I'm protected.* Someone with a belonging wound, like Trish, might communicate passively instead of aggressively based on reading the environment around them. If belonging requires you to be easygoing, then a passive communication style makes sense. You might notice that you use one style with one person and another style with another. But what I really want you to begin to notice is where you go when your wound is under attack and you're trying to protect it and be seen, heard, and understood.

I want us to explore a few things together. Think about any relationship where communication breaks down. Bring only one relationship to focus for now, but you can do this as many times through as you want. I want you to think about which communication style you use when conflict gets activated with this person and just identify it now. Are you passive or aggressive with them, do you find yourself engaging passive-aggressively, or is your style disorganized and a combination of all three? How does that style of communication attempt to protect you?

Next, I want you to take a moment to consider what styles of communication existed in your family system growing up. Is your current style of communication a repetition of or an opposition to that which you observed or experienced? Remember how valuable it was for Trish to see how she was taking a path of opposition? Tune in with yourself here to see if you're attempting something similar.

As you look closer at the relationship you brought into focus, can you identify which wound gets activated when communication breaks down? And how does that wound keep you from clear, direct communication? That constraint question is so important. If Ally was answering this question, she might bring into focus her relationship with her mother and acknowledge that her safety wound gets activated and becomes the constraint to clear, direct communication. She feels she can't be direct or she'll be met with defensiveness and manipulation. If Veronica was speaking, she'd bring into focus her partner and say her worthiness wound is the constraint. She'd try to find proof of commitment through testing rather than through clear, direct communication.

This is great awareness, but it doesn't end here. This awareness must be used to start formulating your needs and communicating them clearly. Moving from emotional reactivity to clear, kind, direct communication is the goal. *What are you actually trying to say?* As I said earlier in this chapter, before you say anything, your goal is to get clear on what you're trying to say, but in order to get clear, you're going to have to peel back some layers. I know that's a lot to consider, it can feel like a lot to think about and process before you say anything, but we are in the homestretch, and if you're going to make some significant changes in your life, you'll need to do some heavy lifting.

The truth is, this is why you do this work here. It *is* too much to do at a point when you're in conversation or conflict. It's pretty hard to excuse yourself in the midst of a conflict and pull out this book and work through the steps. Imagine that! So work on it now. Roll up your sleeves and keep getting to know yourself, your wounds, and your conflict and communication styles. Let your needs become clear to you. The more you know yourself, the easier it is to navigate this in the moment.

YOUR FREEDOM

Years ago I read a quote from Shonda Rhimes, the ever-impressive producer, screenwriter, and author, that summed up to me why communication is so important. Here's what she said: "Because no matter how hard a conversation is, I know that on the other side of that difficult conversation lies peace. Knowledge. An answer delivered. Character is revealed. Truces are formed. Misunderstandings are resolved. Freedom lies across the field of difficult conversations. And the more difficult the conversation, the greater the freedom." On the other side of difficult conversations are answers, an opening for a path forward, and, as Rhimes says, freedom. But I must highlight one thing here. This freedom that she talks about requires your awareness. It requires conscious communication. There isn't a whole lot of freedom if you're passive, aggressive, passive-aggressive, or disorganized. There isn't a whole lot of freedom if the hard conversation you have is with your activated wounds in control and about to go to battle. *That*, my friends, will hold you hostage. Your freedom lies across the field of difficult conversations when you choose to engage differently.

Ally's freedom was on the other side of having a vulnerable conversation that she had previously resisted with the guy she had been dating. Trish's freedom required her to take responsibility for a communication style that was an attempt to keep her safe but instead was pushing others away. Veronica's freedom required her to stop being passive-aggressive and to use her voice to communicate her pain. And Miyako and Jin found more and more freedom each time they had a hard conversation that revealed more of their stories to each other.

Hard conversations don't always garner the results or outcomes that you want, but they always offer you something invaluable. The victory may not mean that the other person heard you, but it may mean that you honored yourself. The victory may not mean that the other person wants to date exclusively, but it may mean that you were vulnerable and expressed yourself, something you rarely do. The victory may not mean that your friends are ready to be close again, but it may mean that you took ownership and apologized for something that you previously would have ignored. You make changes in your communication style because it honors you and others better. You become freer because you choose not to be controlled by the things from the past that used to rule your life. *You* are in charge, and don't you ever forget it.

10

BOUNDARIES

For most of my life, I had terrible boundaries. This probably comes as no shock to you, but in case there's any confusion, pretending to be a woman with no needs is not the recipe for healthy boundaries. I maintained my "cool girl" status by pretending that I was okay with everything. I was convinced that if I set a boundary, it would mean that a partner would leave me or a friend would be disappointed and upset with me. This was intolerable to me. I wanted to preserve relationships at all costs, even at the cost of my own well-being. I wanted to remain connected to people even if that meant disappointing myself or overextending myself. "Connection" was a lifeline, and as long as I made sure all of my relationships were happy with me, I believed I was safe.

There's a line from the poem "The Invitation" by Oriah that reads: "I want to know if you can disappoint another to stay true to yourself." I remember the first time I read that poem and found this sentence. It brought me to tears. *I want to know if you can disappoint another to stay true to yourself.*

Oof. This was not the way I was living. I would disappoint myself before I would disappoint another, I was too afraid of losing my connection to them, even if ultimately that connection was a false one. I was afraid to disappoint people because I grew up being split between two parents—disappointing one of them was always the outcome. I saw the pain, the hurt, and the chaos that it created.

If you remember, my parents went through a nine-year divorce process. When I was just seven years old, I was asked to join the judge in his chambers. The judge said to me, "Hi, Vienna, I'm going to ask you some questions about your parents. Our conversation is going to be recorded and both of your parents are going to get a copy." He proceeded to ask me questions about which parent I enjoyed living with more, which home I preferred, and where I felt the most comfortable. But all I could think was: *My parents are going to hear my answers, so how can I make sure I don't hurt or disappoint either one of them.*

What I was essentially being asked was: *Are you choosing your mom, or are you choosing your dad?* It never dawned upon me that the third option was: *What does it look like to choose yourself?* The fact that this entire process was considered appropriate dumbfounds me, but alas, the terrible boundaries I had as a result of my safety wound were only exacerbated. To be clear, it is never a child's responsibility to have healthy boundaries. It is always the responsibility of the adults to create the environment for healthy boundaries to exist. But in the absence of healthy boundaries, I learned to protect *their* feelings instead of getting curious about mine.

When the adults around you don't have healthy boundaries, you grow up in an environment that teaches you not to have healthy boundaries either. To choose yourself feels too uncomfortable, too foreign, too selfish. But healthy boundaries are not selfish, despite the fact that some argue they are. They're self-loving and self-considerate, yes . . . but they're respectful of other people as well. Those with healthy boundaries are open with those they trust. They don't over-share, they value their own opinions and make room for others, they're clear and direct communicators, comfortable saying no and hearing it without personalizing it, and they honor their values.

As my friend and colleague Nedra Glover Tawwab says, "Boundaries are meant to preserve relationships." They are the invisible line between you and everything that isn't you. It's like having an invisible filtration system that helps you sort through what's okay and what's not okay in relationships. They help you get clear on the rules, expectations, and conditions of a relationship so that you can feel both close and connected to the other person but also safe, protected, and respected. Boundaries help you teach others how you want to be treated, what is acceptable or unacceptable, and they help you match your yeses with your yeses and your noes with your noes so resentment, burnout, frustration, and anger don't take over.

In most scenarios, we want to employ healthy boundaries, but I need to acknowledge up front that there are absolutely moments when protecting yourself is the most important priority. If you are in an abusive dynamic, if you're in an unsafe situation, crossing your boundaries could quite possibly be the thing that saves your life or keeps you safe in a particular moment. What is laid out in this chapter is appropriate when you feel safe in your environment.

Two Types of Unhealthy Boundaries

When I see clients who need help establishing boundaries, they always fall into one of two camps—those whose boundaries are too porous and those whose boundaries are too rigid. Both are unhealthy in different ways, so let's examine each in turn.

POROUS BOUNDARIES

I love the boundary terms that Dr. Alexandra Solomon uses in her book *Loving Bravely*. The first, porous boundaries, was the way I used to engage. I was the poster child for porous boundaries. I was a people pleaser, feared letting others down, couldn't say no, and wanted to make sure everyone was always happy with me. People with porous boundaries often struggle with codependence, overshare, seek out constant validation, and often accept mistreatment to try to stay connected to or in the good graces of another. Porous boundaries are like a broken-down fence. The structure of that fence might still be around your home, but the wood is rotting, it has gaping holes in it, and the door is off its hinges with no lock. Anything can come in and out as it pleases.

People with porous boundaries usually avoid fixing their fence because it risks and threatens something. They're afraid of being disliked. They don't want to disappoint, upset, or let others down. And they struggle to deal with the guilt that others place on them—fearful that if they take a stand, they'll push others away or be seen as difficult. Maybe you have a friend who never takes no for an answer, and you just go along with what she wants so that there isn't conflict. Or maybe you pick up every one of your mother's phone calls no matter where you are or what you're doing to avoid hearing the guilt trip. You'll learn how to work through this later, but for now you might begin to notice which relationships in your life have porous boundaries.

RIGID BOUNDARIES

Alternatively, a person with rigid boundaries is *not* a people pleaser. They tend to avoid intimacy and closeness. They might struggle to open up or ask for help; they might struggle to trust others. Those with rigid boundaries are protective of personal information and avoid vulnerability, and they might have strict rules that seem inflexible and unreasonable.

Remember that porous fence? Think about rigid boundaries as a concrete wall. That concrete wall is so high that no one can even see the home. There's no door or opening. The main job of this wall is to keep people out. There's no way for connection to happen here.

Remember Mark and Troy? Mark's stonewalling is an example of rigid boundaries. He put up that tall concrete wall, and Troy couldn't get ahold of him, contact him, or know when he was returning home. Mark was keeping Troy at a distance to try to protect himself from feeling criticized.

People with rigid boundaries usually avoid dropping their wall because it risks and threatens something. At the core of rigid boundaries is the fear of being hurt. People with rigid boundaries prioritize protecting themselves because their past experiences have taught them that when they let someone get close to them or when they open up, bad things happen.

How Wounds Block Healthy Boundaries

Not wanting people to be upset with you, being afraid of letting people down, feeling worried about being hurt, and not wanting bad things to happen are very convincing reasons to avoid healthy boundaries. But the real reason you avoid healthy boundaries is because your wound is activated.

Can you see how hard it would be to honor your boundaries (or the boundaries of others) when your goal is to establish your worthiness, belonging, prioritization, trust, or safety at all costs? Just think about that for a moment.

- Imagine that your friend has canceled last minute on you a few times in a row. But because your belonging wound is activated and you've learned that the best way to belong is by remaining as likable as possible, you never express how disrespectful it feels.

- Or imagine that a friend tells you she's exhausted and needs to get some sleep, but because your prioritization wound is in the driver's seat, you won't accept no as an answer to avoid feeling unimportant. You tell her she's going to miss a great night out and that you'll be upset with her if she doesn't come.

- Or imagine the person you're dating keeps asking you to open up and talk about how you're feeling, but the last time you opened up to a partner, he broke up with you. Your safety wound predominates, so you keep a rigid boundary and protect yourself.

These are all boundary violations. And your present-day boundary violations were taught to you at one point, either through what you observed, what you experienced, or what was expected of you.

When your wounds are activated, the likelihood of your having porous or rigid boundaries goes up. How does your activated wound block you from having healthy boundaries? Let's get curious here for a moment.

- My wound is _____.
- The way I protect that wound is being _____ with my boundaries (porous or rigid).
- The quick fix this gives me is _____.
- The impact this has on the other person is _____.

HOW INAUTHENTIC CONNECTION BLOCKS COMMUNICATION AND BOUNDARIES

I could tell that something was off just by the look on Ally's face. "Is everything okay?" I asked. "How are things going in the relationship?"

It was still early in the relationship, but I hadn't gotten any updates in a couple of weeks.

"It's okay. I think he might be losing interest. I'm not sure what's going on, but he's been late to our last few dates by, like, thirty minutes each time. I feel embarrassed sitting at the bar by myself waiting for him."

"Oh, Ally, I'm sorry. I can imagine how uncomfortable that could be, and why you would start wondering what's going on. Have you talked to him about this?" I asked.

"No, I don't want to say anything because I don't want to upset him. I just worry that if I say something, it will then mean we'll have to have the conversation and then he'll break up with me."

Ally was prioritizing remaining connected to Mike over communicating what needed to change. She didn't want to risk losing the relationship, so she was bargaining with herself to accept mistreatment. *I'd rather deal with my time not being honored than risk the relationship ending.* She was choosing to preserve the relationship instead of setting a healthy boundary.

In Ally's mind, it was safer for her to internalize everything and pretend everything was fine than to state a healthy boundary and risk conflict and the relationship. She learned to do this with her mother when she was growing up, and she also watched her father do the same thing. He would rather let things slide than get into conflict.

"Ally, he's crossing a boundary of yours, can you see it?" I asked.

"Yes, but he had good reasons. He had to stay late at work one night, another time he had to take his dog out before coming, and another time his mom had called, and she needed help with something. Am I supposed to tell him not to do those things?"

Ally was looking for any excuse in the book to avoid setting a boundary. All of this could have been true, but it didn't change the fact that Ally still needed to communicate the boundary. It would be up to Mike to manage his time better. It would be up to Mike to com-municate earlier, or to organize his day in such a way that would al-low him to honor the date time. Maybe he would need to set the time for thirty minutes later so that he didn't keep Ally waiting. All of that was for Mike to figure out. Of course we get held up at work some-times, of course dogs need to go to the bathroom, and of course it's okay to help family out. None of that is what this is about. Ally needed to move from her porous boundaries (*Let me stay connected to you at all costs*) to healthy boundaries if she wanted a genuinely connected relationship.

Ally already knew that she was avoiding a healthy boundary. But from there I wanted her to identify what she was choosing by main-taining her porous boundary. "What do you think it is?" I asked.

Ally was making sure that Mike wouldn't be upset with her and then leave her. *This* was what became the priority; how she was being treated wasn't important.

As we moved toward setting healthy boundaries, I had to let Ally know that this might also alert her safety wound. When something is unfamiliar to us, it's usually quite destabilizing at first. Even though setting a healthy boundary is objectively a good thing, Ally would experience it as a new thing. And new things are unknown. New things are uncertain. New things can feel risky. She doesn't have any evidence that setting a healthy boundary can work out, so it's no wonder she avoids it.

To move from a porous boundary to a healthy boundary would ask Ally to risk what is ultimately an inauthentic connection in order to honor herself. Healthy boundaries would ask Ally to communicate the impact of Mike's being late to their dates even though she under-stood his intentions were good. Healthy boundaries would ask Ally to bravely step toward self-respect while also honoring and respect-ing Mike.

Even though Ally's safety wound would have preferred her to keep quiet and pretend nothing was wrong so that the relationship wouldn't be risked, her healing would require something different of her. In long-lasting healing, your wounds and healthy boundaries work together.

"What do you think it could sound like?" I asked Ally.

"I guess what I need to say is that I understand that things happen and plans will change, but that I'd like him to respect my time better by being on time. Maybe I could even tell him that it feels embarrassing and disrespectful when he's late?" Ally was trying healthy boundaries out with me as practice.

"That's great," I said. "Your safety wound wants to protect you, but when it's running the show, it doesn't actually protect *you*, it protects what you're afraid of having happen at the expense of you. Do you see that?

"When you don't maintain healthy boundaries for yourself, you aren't authentically connected. You're holding back. You're connected through something inauthentic. Sometimes when you set healthy boundaries, you will lose relationships. I know that's hard to think about, but your goal is to be in relationships that are open, authentic, and truly connected. You don't want the illusion of that. That's not healing."

Moving from Porous to Healthy Boundaries

If you have porous boundaries, I want you to consider what relationships or dynamics in your life have set you up to be a people pleaser. I want you to consider where your fear of letting others down comes from, or why saying no is so hard. What's the story around why you need to make sure everyone is happy, or why you've learned it's okay for people to mistreat you and for you to stay quiet about it? There is a story here, I can promise you that. And from there, I'd encourage you to work through these questions:

	If Ally was to answer those questions, here's what she would have said.
1. What wound is your porous boundary trying to protect?	1. My safety wound.
2. If you replaced it with a healthy boundary, what are you afraid will happen?	2. That my partner will shut down, become defensive, or leave me.
3. What does that fear remind you of?	3. What happened with my mom growing up.
4. What are you choosing to emphasize or prioritize if you maintain a porous boundary?	4. I'm emphasizing staying connected to Mike to make sure he doesn't leave me.
5. Assess what you need to both honor yourself and also feel safe.	5. I want my time to be respected and I also want this relationship to continue.
6. Assess what you think the other person needs in order to honor them and for them to feel respected.	6. I think Mike would want me to know that he means well and that he's not a bad person because of this.
7. Communicate the boundary.	7. Mike, I really love getting to know you and I really enjoy our dates. I would like you to be on time or make our dates for later so that I don't have to wait for you for thirty minutes. It doesn't respect my time.

Guess what happens if she sticks with porous boundaries? She cycles through those first three questions indefinitely. Her safety wound keeps her from setting a healthy boundary, because the fear of what that healthy boundary might do reminds her of something from the past. Do you see it? The fear maintains the porous boundary, and around and around she goes. Around and around *you* go.

Healthy boundaries require you to step out of what you know. Whew. I know it's hard because I've been there, too. But an act of courage can change your course.

MY ACT OF COURAGE

I speak about boundaries from personal experience as well as professional expertise. It took one significant moment in my life to make the shift from porous boundaries to healthy ones. In my late twenties I was dating someone I thought was "the one," but not too long after we had started dating, his ex wanted to get back together with him. He was confused and stressed and didn't know what to do. I was still in my "cool girl" phase, so I told him to take all the time he needed, that I understood how hard this must be on him, and that I'd be happy to support him in what he decided. *If I'm super easygoing, he'll want to be with me, right?* Something like that.

But one day in conversation with a friend, I realized I was repeating my early role from my childhood. I was pretending to be fine with something that I wasn't fine with. He and his ex had seen each other, were talking a lot to figure out whether they'd get back together, and I—still his girlfriend at the time!—was pretending to be unaffected by it. *Don't be too difficult, don't have needs, he might leave you.* It hit me so clearly that day. I was done with the role, and I was done pretending.

I remember the words I spoke to him, the healthy boundary I set that night after weeks of this. I called him and nervously said, "I'm not okay with what you're doing, and how you're handling this is disrespectful and dishonorable to me. You keep thinking that you're trying to choose between me and her, but you have to figure out what it means to choose yourself, and I don't see you doing that. I'm going to make things easier and remove myself from the possibilities for you."

I ended things with him that night and never spoke to him again. Not once. I cried for what seemed like months. It was awful. This was someone I'd thought I had a future with, but the moment I saw how my worthiness wound was keeping me from having healthy boundaries, and the moment I saw how I had carried my role from my family of origin into this relationship was the biggest wake-up call I had ever had. If I had to answer those questions, here is what they would have sounded like:

---

1. What wound is your porous boundary trying to protect?

1. My worthiness wound.

2. If you replaced it with a healthy boundary, what are you afraid will happen?

2. That he will leave me and go back to his ex.

3. What does that fear remind you of?

3. That something or someone is more important than how I'm feeling.

4. What are you choosing to emphasize or prioritize if you maintain a porous boundary?

4. Mistreatment.

5. Assess what you need to both honor yourself and also feel safe.

5. I need to share how disrespectful this is, and I need to become okay with whatever the outcome might be.

6. Assess what you think the other person needs in order to honor them and for them to feel respected.

6. Kindness, thoughtfulness. To see that he's struggling. But I also need to be direct with him.

7. Communicate the boundary.

7. I'm not okay with what you're doing, and how you're handling this is disrespectful and dishonorable to me. You keep thinking that you're trying to choose between me and her, but you have to figure out what it means to choose yourself, and I don't see you doing that. I'm going to make things easier and remove myself from the possibilities for you.

What will be your act of courage when it comes to boundaries? Your relationship with your wound is vital. As you choose to set a healthy boundary, you must witness and acknowledge your wound so that it knows you're taking a risk. But there is a difference between an intentional, aware, considered risk and a reckless risk. Your job is to engage the former.

You already know a lot about your wound. You know a lot about why you have porous boundaries and how those boundaries have protected you from the things that are hard for you to face. But I want you to think about what a healthy boundary would be that would replace that porous boundary. I want you to get intentional about it. I want you to recognize the risk that you're taking, but I also want you to tell me why taking that risk is important to you.

- The porous boundary that I have is _____.
- I want to communicate with a healthy boundary that sounds like _____.
- The risk that I'm taking is _____.
- But I'm taking that risk because _____.
- Regardless of the outcome, the way this benefits my origin wound is _____.

Beautiful work. Look for a moment where you can replace your porous boundary with a healthy one. If you can notice it in the moment, incredible! If you notice it afterward, acknowledge what it could have looked like. You may even be able to anticipate with whom a porous boundary might happen. Think ahead, consider what a healthy boundary might be, and then try implementing it.

Moving from Rigid to Healthy Boundaries

Tony's father was physically abusive toward his mother until Tony got strong enough one day to put an end to it. He had avoided relationships his entire life for fear of losing love and connection as he did with his mother when she dissociated after her abuse.

Tony had met someone a couple of months back and he told me how much he liked this woman. She was smart and interesting, he was very attracted to her, and she was also interested in him. "We've gone on a number of dates which have been nice," he said shyly.

"How's the conversation between the two of you?" I asked.

"Well, she does most of the talking and asks me a lot of questions about myself. It's a lot."

"It sounds like she's wanting to get to know you. How does that feel?"

Tony was aware that he had a hard time getting close to people. He had a wall up around his heart, and he made it hard for others to get in and to get to know him. He also held himself back from getting to know others, rarely asking questions. He was guarded. That guard was up for a good reason, but it was also keeping him from partnership, connection, and healing.

"Honestly, it feels hard. It feels heavy. I even feel reactive when she asks me questions about my family, but I guess because we've been working together, I know that it's just pressing on my wound."

This was an incredible insight from Tony. I was impressed with his ability to both feel what he was feeling but also become the observer of himself.

"What do you think opening up a little bit would feel like?" I asked.

"Probably like death," he said. "But I think I have to try. I don't want to stay behind these walls forever. I know that I'll never get close to anyone if I don't. I'll never love. I'll never have authentic connection. I'll never have partnership. Or if I do, I'll always be disappointing the other person. If I just stay like this, it's like my dad wins. It's kind of strange, but I feel like in some ways, me breaking through these walls is me also taking a stand. Like you robbed something from my mom, but you're not going to rob this from me, too. Does that make sense?" he asked.

It did. What Tony was saying was profound. Intentionally coming out from behind that wall was part of his healing. Coming out from behind that wall was his own version of setting a boundary with his father. *I won't let you take love and connection from me. I won't let you keep me from prioritizing relationships for myself or prioritizing opening up to others.* We worked through the same questions:

1. What wound is your rigid boundary trying to protect?
2. If you replaced it with a healthy boundary, what are you afraid will happen?
3. What does that fear remind you of?
4. What are you choosing to emphasize or prioritize if you maintain a rigid boundary?
5. Assess what you need to both honor yourself and also feel safe.
6. Assess what you think the other person needs in order to honor them and for them to feel respected.
7. Safely lift the boundary.

His answers were quick. "It's trying to protect my safety wound. I'm afraid that if I open up and let her in, then my feelings will grow and then she might leave, and I'll be heartbroken. It reminds me of what happened with my mom. I'm choosing to emphasize protecting myself from the possibility of pain. But what I need is to take a risk for love. What she needs is for me to open up. And lifting the boundary safely means that I try sharing one thing first to see how that goes and then maybe I open up a little bit more from there."

Moving from rigid boundaries to healthy boundaries is a gradual shift. It's about taking small steps in the direction of opening up, of sharing yourself with someone you trust.

I rarely hear people in conversations about boundaries talking about the rigid ones—certainly not to the extent that I hear people talking about porous ones. Most social media memes on the topic tend to emphasize setting boundaries and say very little about lifting boundaries. But *lifting* boundaries is just as important. This, too, is an act of courage. This shift from a rigid boundary to a healthy boundary won't ask you to swing the door wide open. Tony wasn't going to share his whole life story all in one shot or pour his heart out and take off all his emotional armor. This shift would be a gradual one.

When you begin to lift a boundary, do it slowly, bit by bit. Remember that healthy boundaries still prioritize protection; they just don't prioritize protection *over* connection. Tony's goal was to figure out the right mix of protection and connection. If you're starting to drop a wall, you're allowed to drop it 5 percent and see what that feels like. If you're starting to build a strong fence, you're allowed to put 10 percent of it up and see what type of protection that offers. You don't need to demolish your whole wall and you don't need to build a fort around you.

There's no perfect recipe for this, but I recommend starting off by sharing just one thing with someone you really trust and seeing how that goes before opening up more or trying it with others. Take the path of least resistance: Share something that isn't too near and dear to your heart. You'll want to choose something that if a person responds negatively toward it, this won't be devastating to you.

Unhealthy boundaries put you on a merry-go-round where healing can't happen. You might notice that you lean toward porous boundaries or that you lean toward rigid boundaries, but you might also notice that you go back and forth or that you engage certain boundaries with certain people. Our boundary style can be person-specific. Whatever you're noticing about yourself and your relationships, it's time to step out of the cycle, move away from the illusion of the quick fix, and slowly implement the boundaries that will show your wound that your worthiness, belonging, prioritization, trust, and safety do not require you to live a life without any protection or with a false connection. You can feel safe and authentically connected, and in healthy dynamics, others will not just support that, they'll celebrate that with you.

PART IV

YOUR RECLAMATION

11

MAKING IT STICK

As we partner, maintain friendships, and become parents, we will almost certainly notice the ways we've repeated the wounds we experienced in our own childhoods. Our parents' wounds become our
wounds, which in turn become our children's wounds. This is normal,
but not inevitable. Interrupting that pattern (or at least recognizing it)
is the work of this book and the work of a lifetime. You *can* forge a new
path forward. But the key to this is understanding your origin stories
and making conscious choices about how to integrate that knowledge
and move ahead into a new future. Otherwise the twin demons—
repetition and opposition—will still run the show.

When I describe repetition and opposition to my clients, I have
them visualize a pendulum swinging. So many of us veer from one
extreme to the other, repeating our patterns or flailing against them,
on and on, mindlessly. But when you're swinging, you're not in control; you're in chaos. That's no way to live. There's a different way:
integration.

Integration is the center point of the pendulum, where the weighted
balls come together and stop their out-of-control movement. Integration lives in the space between the two reactive extremes. This is where
you get to experience stillness, calm, and grounding. You reach

integration by getting to know your origin wounds, spending time with your pain, and processing the messages you received and the meaning you attached to them.

Integration is a practice in which you bring the parts of the self together. You match the outside with the inside. Your decisions align with your truth and what's authentic for you. The way that you act and treat people is in line with your authentic self instead of your wounded self. Instead of being led by fear, insecurity, or unhealed origin wounds, you can put into action the behaviors that support your goals.

Here's more good news: Change can happen. I don't need any research to support this. I *know* this because I have the great honor of working with people day in and day out who show me this. But we've also seen this proven through neuroplasticity, the brain's ability to change. And although this rewiring and reorganizing is easier when we are younger, it's still available to us as adults. Studies have shown that neuroplasticity gets enhanced when we do daily physical exercise, increasing the blood flow to the brain, and when we learn new things and pay attention. That's why staying open and curious through this work is so life-changing.

If you're still here, you're doing it. You have had to stay open throughout this book. You've looked at yourself, your stories, your beliefs, and your experiences through a new lens. You've acknowledged things about yourself that might not have been easy to acknowledge, and you've seen your part in your unhealthy patterns. *You*, my friend, are doing life-changing work, truly.

You've probably figured out by now that you're the only one who is in charge of your change. You get to choose how you respond, how you engage in conflict, how you communicate, and what boundaries you set and lift. How others respond to that is not in your control, and if you wait for them to make the first move, you might be waiting a very long time.

I don't want you to underestimate the work involved. Relational habits that you've been repeating for decades are automatic. They're waiting for the moment you lack awareness, the moment you look the other way so that they can repeat the same old patterns. Before you even know it, you're right back at the same reaction, the same conflict, and the same passive-aggressive communication style. That's why you can read a book like this, do the exercises, nod in agreement throughout the chapters, and have your own oof moments that resonate deeply and still find yourself back in autopilot mode in just a few short weeks.

Frustrating, I know.

But it's also okay. I want to remind you that you're not going to transform overnight. Integration is a mindset, but it's also a process. It doesn't happen all at once, but bit by bit, piece by piece. You will practice one small shift again and again. And then another and another. And those small shifts create bigger shifts. I am reminded of a quote from Lionel Messi, the Argentinian footballer, who is considered one of the greatest to ever live. He says, "I start early and I stay late, year after year. It took me 17 years and 114 days to become an overnight success." If you set yourself up with unachievable goals when the small stuff hasn't been practiced, you will feel like you're failing and lose confidence in yourself. Your victories are in the process.

Doing this work is vital not only to the quality of your relationships but also to your overall health. We know that adults in satisfying partnerships are physically and emotionally healthier than those in unhappy relationships. But it's not just about partnership. One of the longest-running studies to date, out of Harvard University, shows that those most satisfied in their relationships, any relationship, at age fifty were the healthiest at age eighty. George Vaillant, the Harvard psychiatrist who directed the study from 1972 to 2004, said that there are two foundational elements to this: "One is love. The other is finding a way of coping with life that does not push love away." Whew. There's a lot of incentive to make space for love and to recognize what keeps you from it or what blocks it.

How do you make room for authentic love? How do you make room for connection? How can you safely create space for intimacy? And how do you stop engaging in the things that block all of that or push it away? You've done a beautiful job exploring these questions already and you know that your unresolved origin wounds have a lot to do with moving you forward.

Whether you know it or not, you've already begun the process of making room for authentic love, connection, and intimacy in your partnerships, friendships, and familial relationships just by picking up this book and exploring these pages. But if you want it to stick, you'll have to commit to a lifelong practice.

This isn't meant to be intimidating. Quite the contrary. I think it would be way harder to carry the pressure of figuring it out and implementing it all right away. What I'm telling you is that you have a lifetime of figuring it out. You have a lifetime of becoming more and more aware in moments and responding differently, regulating yourself, and navigating through conflict with different goals in mind. They're in the moment you recognize that you are being passive-aggressive and choose to stop and communicate differently. They're in the moment that you take ownership for something you'd normally defend. And they're in the moment when you remind yourself that being authentic is more important than having someone validate your inauthenticity.

I'm also telling you the process of becoming more aware is well worth it. Awareness without accountability is just knowledge. You can't rely on your knowledge alone to live a life of authenticity, ease, and peace. Awareness with accountability is wisdom. This is where growth happens. Integration doesn't happen without wisdom.

Leading with Authenticity

If you have made a habit out of trading authenticity for attachment, or even if you only do it from time to time, then part of this work is about reclaiming your authenticity. This isn't an easy task in a world that is constantly asking you to prioritize everything else over your true self, but it's a challenge worth accepting. This challenge asks you to build confidence in your own worthiness, belonging, prioritization, safety, and trust instead of believing that you must change who you are in order to get that from others.

Our families of origin are often where we engage in the first forms of self-abandonment. As you've learned, there can be a lot of spoken and unspoken pressure to leave who you are, to abandon or betray your authentic self to essentially take care of another. Sometimes this takes place quite literally, and other times this caretaking happens by altering yourself so there's less reactivity, anger, stress, or disappointment from the adults around you. But your job was never to manage the emotional experience of others; it was always their responsibility to be in charge of themselves. I'm sorry if you had to do that for them or walk a tightrope when you were around them. But you also have agency in your life now. Just to be clear, I'm not suggesting that you don't care about others. I'm suggesting that you don't take on the burden of processing their emotions for them while you lose yourself and your authenticity. Let that sink in.

To lead with authenticity will require you to stop bending yourself. It will ask you to stop the repetition of what you learned to do long ago and focus your energy on your authenticity. Take a moment to consider the ways you bend yourself today so that you are chosen, accepted, validated, or loved. Have you ever asked any of these questions: *Who do I need to be in order to get this person to want to be with me? To stay with me? To love me? To choose me? To prioritize me?* Do you feel like you need to pretend in any way? Do you focus more on who you think the other person wants you to be instead of connecting to who you are? These questions might feel disturbing to ask and answer. But the answers (or sometimes just asking the questions) will reveal the learned behaviors you adopted years ago in order to survive and attempt getting your needs met, behaviors that are no longer necessary. What you once needed to do to create a sense of worthiness or belonging, to be prioritized, or to establish trust or safety for yourself may be the exact thing that keeps you from the relationships you desire. This is a big part of the work: to see what it is you'd like to keep, and to begin to shed what no longer serves you.

Of course we want someone to want us, to stay with us, to love us, and to choose us. But the ways we've learned to get what we want actually make it *harder* for us to achieve our desired outcome. You see, when you're shapeshifting or performing for love, you'll never know whether what's being given is because of the real you or the you you've learned to present. The only way to trust what's being given is by being yourself. This might not be revolutionary, but it still packs a punch.

I want to be clear here that choosing yourself does not mean being selfish. Choosing yourself means honoring your authenticity. It means being able to stand with your head held high and speak your truth without betraying yourself for others. This is hard. Really, really hard, especially when the consequence is being judged, shamed, rejected, or even disowned. But when you arrive at this place, a sense of calm will wash over you, the discovery of a hard but liberating truth: *It's actually okay if you don't agree, if you criticize me, or even mock me. I know that this is true for me, and because of that I experience freedom by belonging to myself.* Whew. Sovereignty of Self is birthed; it is not automatic.

When you trade authenticity for attachment, it exposes a wound. You are revealing a desire for your wound to be temporarily relieved by others. Your fear of not belonging is relieved when you say something you don't believe just to fit in. Your fear of not being worthy of love is relieved when you pretend that you're okay with things you're not okay with just to not upset a partner. You outsource temporary relief instead of tending to it yourself to establish permanent relief.

It's important to surround yourself with as many people as possible who do not ask you to be inauthentic. Of course that might not be your reality right now, but over time that is the shift you're aiming for. And note that sometimes the person you surround yourself with who asks you to be the most inauthentic is you. (I had to leave a few oofs for the end.) Might you gently identify who in your life asks you to be something other than who you are? And might you explore for a moment what you get from trading your authenticity?

Everything you've done so far in the book has led you to this moment. If leading with authenticity still feels hard, then that lets you know the wound is still too raw for you to do that. Instead of getting frustrated with yourself, remain curious. You will always know deep down what you need to know. You may need to learn to decipher the signals your body sends you, but information is being revealed to you constantly.

But if you're ready to give authenticity a shot, then a good place to start is by identifying where in your life you give it up the most. Is it when you want to fit in? When you want to belong to a group? Is it with a parent? Is it with one of your friends? On a date? We've done a lot of work to identify the origin wounds, but now you need to scan your relationships and your environment to see where you're still being asked to be inauthentic. Choose one relationship for now and think about how you trade authenticity for worthiness, belonging, prioritization, safety, or trust. Do you pretend to like something on a date that you don't, just to impress the other person? Do you go along with something that has always made you feel uncomfortable just to make it easy for your family? Notice what you do.

My challenge for you is to replace one inauthentic moment with an authentic one. Take the risk. Try this out when it's low stakes and see how it feels. Notice the moments when you're tempted, notice the moments when you choose inauthenticity, and then come back around to them when you have some space and consider what you could have done, or how you could have responded to honor authenticity.

Living your authenticity won't be something you master in one moment, but you can strengthen it in each moment you recognize that there is a choice between being authentic and being inauthentic, between prioritizing someone else at the expense of yourself and prioritizing and honoring yourself. You're slowing yourself down enough to be able to recognize that there is a choice present, one where you implement what you've learned about yourself and others and begin the practice of making it stick.

Respect the Pause

I always found it annoying when people would tell me to count to ten before responding. I'd start at one and I'd get more pissed every second that would go by. The problem was that I had no idea what to do with that time. I didn't know where to focus my energy, and how to utilize it in a productive and helpful way.

A well-known quote attributed to Viktor Frankl, a Holocaust survivor, author, and psychiatrist, goes like this: "Between stimulus and response there is a space. In that space is our power to choose our response. In our response lies our growth and our freedom." And although there are of course things that make this much more complicated than simply just choosing differently, especially for those navigating trauma or complex trauma, that space he talks about is where we learn how to respect the pause.

The pause is where you notice a wound that's activated. The pause is where you choose to self-regulate by going for a walk, listening to calming music, moving your body, breathing with intention, or asking for a hug from someone whom you trust. The pause is where you remind yourself of what you know about the pattern you find yourself in. The pause is where you begin to ask yourself questions like: *What's familiar about this? What's the origin story here? How do I normally respond? What opportunity is in front of me? What is something healing I can offer myself right now?* and *What is one shift I can make to step out of the cycle?*

The pause is where awareness has a moment to enter. And now that you've read this book, you know where to look. You now know that your reactivity is pointing you to something that's still raw. Instead of engaging and finding yourself right back at the same cycle, you have an opportunity to become curious about yourself. The pause gives you the space to tend to wounds, to identify something, to witness and grieve, and to eventually pivot.

You won't be able to do all of that in a split second. But you might be able to say that you need a moment to process on your own, you might be able to choose to listen and not engage, and eventually you might be able to walk through what's coming up for you with that other person there, deepening the relationship.

Can you think about the last argument or fight you had? It doesn't matter who it was with, just bring it into focus. Do you remember what set you off and how you reacted? And now I want you to visualize the moment before you reacted. If you pretend to take a television remote and literally press pause and see the still image in front of you, that's what I want you to do. And now I want you to notice, inspect, and analyze that still image. What do you see? What's happening?

Who's upset and how do you know? What does your body language give away? What does theirs? And now, in this paused moment, I want you to think about what you would do in this moment now. With everything you know about your wounds, what do you want to offer yourself in that pause? How can you lovingly tend to and honor yourself? I'd encourage you to reflect on this. You can journal about it, you can close your eyes and walk yourself through it, and you might even choose to share these reflections with someone else.

The more you respect the pause, the better you get at it. I will also remind you that your practice usually happens when you're not actually in the game. You might not notice that pause when you're heated. You might notice it and still tell it to screw off. Or you might notice it but not have enough perspective when you're in it. You can build this muscle after the fact. You often have to.

Look back at fights, ruptures, and your reactivity, and reflect: *If I could have respected the pause, what would I have learned about myself? What wound would I have seen activated? Does my reaction match the circumstances in front of me right now? And how could I engage differently, in a way that would be healing?*

The more you respect the pause, the more you honor the space between stimulus and response, as Frankl suggests, the more you can move toward the changes you want for yourself and your relationships. It's in this space where you have a choice between offering yourself peace or experiencing familiar pain. When we start to learn how to utilize this space well, it moves us toward our healing and our freedom.

Peace Versus Suffering

From all of my work, I've learned that most people do not enjoy suffering. That's probably true for you, too. And I might be going out on

264

a limb here, but if you're reading this book, it's probably fair to say that you're interested in minimizing your suffering and pain as much as possible.

When I learned to respect the pause, one of the most helpful prompts for me was, *Is what I'm about to say or do going to lead me to peace or lead me to suffering?* But before we get too deep into your response, you must get clear on how you define peace and suffering. What do these words mean to you? What do they feel like in your body?

The truth is, your decision for peace might not always feel easy or be without discomfort, and suffering might actually feel like the simpler path, one without tension or friction in the moment. Think about this: If prioritizing peace means choosing authenticity but also means that you get rejected, then that choice might feel pretty undesirable and uncomfortable for you. That's what makes this work tricky. But we're not talking about the short term, we're talking about where we want to be headed in the long term. Let's make that question even more focused: *Is what I'm about to do or say going to lead me to suffering or peace within the context of my origin wound healing and expansion goals?*

You might not always be able to choose peace over suffering. In fact, let's set the bar very low. If you can bring an ounce of awareness to your decisions at first, that will be a major victory. Decisions that support your healing do come up against some resistance. That's to be expected.

But at some point, you will replace suffering with peace, even when it feels hard, uncomfortable, and undesirable. The key is to tune into yourself and identify what it is that you're choosing and why you're choosing it. You will feel empowered enough to try on the discomfort because engaging differently and taking accountability for your healing will be an act of self-respect and self-love.

Self-Love

What do you think of when you hear the word *self-love*? I used to confuse this with self-care. I thought self-love was just enjoying massages or bubble baths, going out into nature, and doing things to restore myself. *This* can absolutely be a part of self-love, but when I took time to really sit with how I would define it, I came to this definition. Self-love is the intersection of compassion, grace, and kindness for the self and accountability for, ownership of, and responsibility for the self. One without the other doesn't work. You can't love yourself without making space to see yourself as a flawed human being, allowed to make mistakes and stumble. There must be grace there. But you also can't love yourself if you avoid where you need to take responsibility. You can't love yourself if you're dodging accountability.

You are messy, just like me. You are flawed and deserving. You will make mistakes, you'll let people down, and you'll disappoint others, and you'll still be a worthy human being. But your messiness, it needs your accountability. When you make mistakes, when you let people down and disappoint them, when you hurt others, taking accountability and ownership is one of the most loving things you offer not only others but yourself. When you avoid it, you are telling yourself that your worthiness, belonging, prioritization, safety, and trust are still tied to your perfection. When you avoid it, you teach yourself that there's no room to be both human and loved.

In your integration practice, you will need self-love. You will come face-to-face with your messy human self. You might become upset or frustrated with yourself when you find yourself in an old pattern. You might become ashamed of yourself when you engage in an old behavior you have worked hard at replacing. In these moments especially, you will need to remind yourself that self-love requires both. Both kindness and accountability. Both grace and ownership. Both compassion and responsibility.

Your healing is a work in progress, and it needs you to make space for the very human experience you will have alongside of it. You will become an overnight success decades from now. Chin up. You are doing the most beautiful work that exists; you are participating in your own healing.

CONCLUSION

As you come face-to-face with the pain you've experienced, you'll also come face-to-face with the ways you've contributed to the pain of others. Maybe you haven't prioritized your partner. Maybe you have been critical of your son. Maybe you have been passive-aggressive with your friend. Remember, kindness and accountability. Grace and ownership. Compassion and responsibility. Nothing good comes from being unkind to yourself. Lead with your self-love.

When we become aware of our own shortcomings, it can feel overwhelmingly emotional. Be gentle. Remember, you are a link in a multigenerational system. You've been hurt, wounded, let down, and disappointed. But you've also been the person who has hurt, wounded, let down, and disappointed others. This is what happens. As the old saying goes, "Hurt people, hurt people." But healing people help heal people, too. And even though you can't change anyone else, the healing shifts that you make reverberate through the systems you're in. When you make a change, the change is felt. It might not be liked, but it will undoubtedly be experienced.

You, my friend, are shaking the system. You are stepping out of the old roles you no longer need to fill. You're challenging the beliefs, values, and identity that were given to you from those who came before. You are beginning to choose what it is that *you* believe. You are tending to your wounds, slowing down to witness and grieve with them. Giving them the proper attention and care that they've needed. They'll make an appearance from time to time, but when they do, you'll know what to do.

You are changing the way you relate to conflict and making space for it to lead you to connection, to healing, and to a deep sense of intimacy between you and the other person. You are changing the way you communicate, replacing the old ways that maintain your wounds with clear, direct, and kind communication that honors you and the other person. You are giving yourself permission to set boundaries, even when it feels uncomfortable. You are beginning to lift boundaries, to give connection and closeness another shot. To believe that there are people in the world who can be close to you without taking advantage of you, without hurting you, or without using you. You are beginning to do all of this because you opened yourself up to explore your family, your origin stories, and origin wounds.

My friend, this work that you're doing, it's remarkable. You are brave and courageous; you are strength embodied. You are choosing to pick up the pieces and create a new path forward for yourself. Although you and I have worked through this book without being face-to-face with each other, I can't tell you how proud I am of you. I know what goes into the work that you've just done. Everything I've asked you to do here, I've asked of myself. This is some serious heavy lifting, and you're doing it.

I hope that you've learned something new about yourself in our work together. I hope that by delving into your origin stories you've gained new perspective. I hope that you've seen yourself and others through a new lens. And even though you probably started reading this book for you as the adult child, you may have noticed yourself reading it as a partner, as a friend, or even as a parent yourself. You may have seen yourself in some of the stories shared in this book, but you also may have seen your parent, your partner, your sibling, or your friend in one of the stories, too. What a beautiful reminder that we all have a story that most people know very little about.

And what a gift that is to be able to think about anyone that way, but especially the people you care about and love. To remind yourself that they were a child once, too, that they grew up in an imperfect family, one that likely impacted them and left wounds. There's an exercise that author and researcher Dr. Michael Kerr offers that helps us shift to filial maturity, the perspective of seeing one's parents as real people, individuals in their own right, not just as Mommy or Daddy. He asks us to "think of your mother as your grandmother's daughter, and get to know her that way."

And imagine if you can continue to see yourself that way, too. Remind yourself that in all of your painful and frustrating moments, there is a story present, one that is rich with history, one that wants your attention, one worth spending time with. I hope you'll continue to get to know your origin stories. There's always more that can be revealed to you.

ACKNOWLEDGMENTS

Writing this book was one of my greatest professional challenges. I'm a big believer that in order to write about people's stories, to write about relationships, and to write about healing, you must have an intimate relationship with your own story and with others' stories as well.

I am so grateful for every human who has ever asked me to walk alongside them in the therapeutic space. To my clients, past and present, I have learned so much from you. It is one of my greatest honors to get to know your stories and to be with you through the ebb and flow of healing. Thank you for showing up, for opening up, and for always inspiring me. So much of my belief in people's capacity for change comes from watching you bravely make shifts in your lives, large and small.

To my professors, supervisors, advisors, colleagues, and clinicians I've learned from near and far: Thank you for inspiring, teaching, and guiding with grace. I will always remain a student.

To my agents, Steve Troha and Jan Bauer: Thank you for the gentle push. Thank you for doing whatever it took to have me write this book. I found that there was just a bit of magic on the other side of dropping in and getting to it.

To my editor, Michelle Howry: It's a funny thing to say, but I knew it was you from the moment I met you. Your excitement, dedication, vision, and hard work are easy to spot. You are kind, thoughtful, and intentional, the type of person and energy with which I like to keep close company. Thank you for your brilliance.

To Dedi: WE did it. I am certain I could not have done this without you. Thank you for your patience, guidance, vision, and hard work. I'm so glad we could find humor through this process. We kept each other going and I am forever grateful to have had you as a guide and support for my first book. This book is better because of you.

To my team at Penguin Random House: Thank you for your creative vision, support, and dedication. There is so much that happens behind the scenes to bring books alive, and I am forever grateful to all of you for the endless things that often get overlooked.

To Alexandra and Angelica: Thank you for taking a look at this manuscript when I needed eyes on it. I am so grateful for your feedback.

To every single soul helper of mine: Thank you for holding up a mirror to me to activate change. Some of you know who you are, but many more of you have no idea of the impact you've had or the healing that has happened once our chapter closed. I acknowledge you and appreciate you.

To my dear friends: Thank you for the love and encouragement always, and especially through this process. You are my family, my sisters and brothers, and writing this book would have been way less enjoyable without you checking in on me, laughing with me, and crying with me.

To my parents: You both gave me so much, even when it was hard. I am forever grateful for the love, attention, validation, care, concern, and commitment. Thank you for always encouraging me, and for finding the openings for your own healing and change. You have taught me that things don't stay the same, that chapters end, and that no matter your age, new ways of being and existing can emerge.

ACKNOWLEDGMENTS

To my husband, Connor, my absolute greatest soul helper. You finally got me to write a book! Thank you for seeing where I can go often before I can. Two years ahead, always. You've shown me parts of myself I couldn't see, and you've walked alongside me with the same goals in mind. Thank you for witnessing me, grieving with me, and encouraging my pivots. You have inspired me to change my life in every way that is good. I love you.

NOTES

Introduction: My Family of Origin and Yours

7 **on Integrative Systemic Therapy:** William M. Pinsof, Douglas C. Breulin, William P. Russell, et al., *Integrative Systemic Therapy: Metaframeworks for Problem Solving with Individuals, Couples, and Families* (Washington, DC: American Psychological Association, 2018).

1. Your Past Is Your Present

19 **"The Power of Vulnerability":** Brené Brown, "The Power of Vulnerability," filmed January 3, 2011, at TEDxHouston, Houston, TX, video, 13:04, https://www.youtube.com/watch?v=iCvmsMzlF7o.

19 **in a multigenerational chain:** Mona D. Fishbane, "Differentiation and Dialogue in Intergenerational Relationships," in *Handbook of Clinical Family Therapy,* ed. Jay L. Lebow (Hoboken, NJ: John Wiley & Sons, 2005), 543–68.

26 **"attachment trumps authenticity":** Gabor Maté, "Authenticity vs. Attachment," filmed May 14, 2019, video, 4:18, https://www.youtube.com/watch?v=l3bynimi8HQ.

3. I Want to Feel Worthy

64 **course of their lives:** Patricia A. Thomas, Hui Liu, and Debra Umberson, "Family Relationships and Well-Being," *Innovation in Aging* 1, no. 3 (2017): igx025, doi: 10.1093/geroni/igx025.

64 **more vulnerable to depression:** David Denning Luxton, "The Effects of Inconsistent Parenting on the Development of Uncertain Self-Esteem and Depression Vulnerability" (PhD dissertation, University of Kansas, 2017), 86.

4. I Want to Belong

90 **what he calls *horizontals*:** Andrew Solomon, *Far from the Tree: Parents, Children, and the Search for Identity* (New York: Scribner, 2013), 2.

95   **increase in incivility:** Ashley A. Anderson, Dominique Brossard, Dietram
A. Scheufele, et al., "The 'Nasty Effect': Online Incivility and Risk Perceptions
of Emerging Technologies," *Journal of Computer-Mediated Communication*
19, no. 3 (2014): 373–87, doi: 10.1111/jcc4.12009.

95   **ever been before:** Alan I. Abramowitz and Kyle L. Saunders, "Is Polariza-
tion a Myth?," *The Journal of Politics* 70, no. 2 (2008): 542–55, doi: 10.1017/
s0022381608080493.

97   **cultural knowledge, and appearance:** W. S. Carlos Poston, "The Biracial
Identity Development Model: A Needed Addition," *Journal of Counseling &
Development* 69, no. 2 (1990): 152–55, doi: 10.1002/j.1556-6676.1990
.tb01477.x.

98   **what gets acknowledgment:** William E. Cross Jr., *Shades of Black: Diver-
sity in African-American Identity* (Philadelphia: Temple University Press,
1991), 39–74.

102 **relationships with others:** David Morris Schnarch, "Differentiation: Developing a Self-in-Relation," in *Passionate Marriage: Love, Sex, and Intimacy
in Emotionally Committed Relationships* (New York: W. W. Norton, 2009),
53–74.

104 **"sacrificing who we are":** Brené Brown, *Braving the Wilderness: The Quest
for True Belonging and the Courage to Stand Alone* (New York: Random
House, 2017), 37.

5. I Want to Be Prioritized

113 *covert expectations:* Robert A. Glover, *No More Mr. Nice Guy! A Proven
Plan for Getting What You Want in Love, Sex, and Life* (Philadelphia: Running Press, 2003).

121 **generation to generation:** Susan Branje, Sanne Geeraerts, Eveline L. de
Zeeuw, et al., "Intergenerational Transmission: Theoretical and Method-
ological Issues and an Introduction to Four Dutch Cohorts," *Developmental
Cognitive Neuroscience* 45 (2020): 100835, doi: 10.1016/j.dcn.2020.10085.

124 **meaning as a couple:** Hannah Eaton, "The Gottman Institute," *The Gottman Institute* (blog), accessed May 30, 2022, https://www.gottman.com/
blog/redefining-individuality-and-togetherness-during-quarantine/.

125 **needs for autonomy and personal growth:** Eli J. Finkel, Elaine O. Cheung,
Lydia F. Emery, et al., "The Suffocation Model: Why Marriage in America
Is Becoming an All-or-Nothing Institution," *Current Directions in Psycho-
logical Science* 24, no. 3 (2015): 238–44, doi: 10.1177/0963721415569274.

128 **experience one without the other:** Jandy Nelson, *The Sky Is Everywhere*
(New York: Dial Books, 2010), 257.

131 **authoring ones that aren't:** Mary Etchison and David M. Kleist, "Review
of Narrative Therapy: Research and Utility," *The Family Journal* 8, no. 1
(2000): 61–66, doi: 10.1177/1066480700081009.

131 **book *Rising Strong*:** Brené Brown, *Rising Strong: How the Ability to Reset
Transforms the Way We Live, Love, Parent, and Lead* (New York: Random
House, 2017), 90–91.

NOTES

6. I Want to Trust

147 **Strange Situation study:** Mary D. Salter Ainsworth and Silvia M. Bell, "Attachment, Exploration, and Separation: Illustrated by the Behavior of One-Year-Olds in a Strange Situation," *Child Development* 41, no. 1 (1970): 49–67, doi: 10.2307/1127388.

147 **insecure attachment relationships:** Patty X. Kuo, Ekjyot K. Saini, Elizabeth Tengelitsch, et al., "Is One Secure Attachment Enough? Infant Cortisol Reactivity and the Security of Infant-Mother and Infant-Father Attachments at the End of the First Year," *Attachment & Human Development* 21, no. 5 (2019): 426–44, doi: 10.1080/14616734.2019.1582595.

7. I Want to Feel Safe

159 **control over another:** REACH Team, "6 Different Types of Abuse," *REACH Beyond Domestic Violence* (blog), accessed May 30, 2022, https://reachma .org/blog/6-different-types-of-abuse/.

159 **their eighteenth birthday:** Catherine Townsend and Alyssa A. Rheingold, *Estimating a Child Sexual Abuse Prevalence Rate for Practitioners: A Review of Child Sexual Abuse Prevalence Studies* (Charleston, S.C.: Darkness to Light, 2013), https://www.d2l.org/wp-content/uploads/2017/02/PREVA LENCE-RATE-WHITE-PAPER-D2L.pdf.

160 **denigrate their victims:** Ann Pietrangelo, "Emotional Abuse: What It Is and Signs to Watch For," ed. Jacquelyn Johnson, Healthline (Healthline Media, January 28, 2022), https://www.healthline.com/health/signs-of -mental-abuse.

165 **body and thoughts:** *Diagnostic and Statistical Manual of Mental Disorders: DSM-5*, 5th ed. (Washington, DC: American Psychiatric Association, 2013).

165 **adaptive dissociative experiences:** Janina Fisher, "Dissociative Phenomena in the Everyday Lives of Trauma Survivors," paper presented at the Boston University Medical School Psychological Trauma Conference, Boston, May 2001, https://janinafisher.com/pdfs/dissociation.pdf.

165 **"knowing and not knowing":** Bessel A. van der Kolk, *The Body Keeps the Score: Brain, Mind, and Body in the Healing of Trauma* (New York: Penguin Books, 2015), 123.

174 **pain you're feeling:** Van der Kolk, *The Body Keeps the Score.*

179 **go hand in hand:** Alexandra H. Solomon, *Loving Bravely: 20 Lessons of Self-Discovery to Help You Get the Love You Want* (Oakland, CA: New Harbinger Publications, 2017), 223.

179 **Embodied self-regulation:** Catherine P. Cook-Cottone, "Embodied Self-Regulation," in *Mindfulness and Yoga for Self-Regulation: A Primer for Mental Health Professionals* (New York: Springer Publishing Company, 2015), 3–18.

180 **"what happened to you":** *The Wisdom of Trauma*, directed by Maurizio Benazzo and Zaya Benazzo, featuring Gabor Maté (Science and Nonduality, 2021), https://thewisdomoftrauma.com.

8. Conflict

189 **"Horsemen of the Apocalypse":** John M. Gottman with Nan Silver, "The Four Horsemen of the Apocalypse: Warning Signs," in *Why Marriages Succeed or Fail: And How You Can Make Yours Last* (New York: Simon & Schuster, 1995), 68–102.

196 **"over emotional disconnection":** Susan M. Johnson, *Hold Me Tight: Seven Conversations for a Lifetime of Love* (New York: Little, Brown Spark, 2008), 30.

196 **fear of losing connection:** Johnson, *Hold Me Tight*, 31.

200 **of relational failure:** John M. Gottman, *The Marriage Clinic: A Scientifically Based Marital Therapy* (New York: W. W. Norton, 1999).

205 **reactivity to reflectivity:** Michele Scheinkman and Mona DeKoven Fishbane, "The Vulnerability Cycle: Working with Impasses in Couple Therapy," *Family Process* 43, no. 3 (2004): 279–99, doi: 10.1111/j.1545-5300.2004 .00023.x.

9. Communication

210 **"when you feel upset":** Alexandra H. Solomon, *Loving Bravely: 20 Lessons of Self-Discovery to Help You Get the Love You Want* (Oakland, CA: New Harbinger Publications, 2017), 134.

234 **"the greater the freedom":** Shonda Rhimes, *Year of Yes: How to Dance It Out, Stand in the Sun and Be Your Own Person* (New York: Simon & Schuster Paperbacks, 2015), 225.

10. Boundaries

236 **"stay true to yourself":** Oriah, *The Invitation* (San Francisco: HarperSanFrancisco, 1999), 2.

238 **"meant to preserve relationships":** Nedra Glover Tawwab (@nedratawwab), "Set Boundaries, Find Peace," Instagram Live, March 8, 2022, https://www .instagram.com/tv/Ca2rtM0lwKl/.

238 **book *Loving Bravely*:** Alexandra H. Solomon, "Establish Healthy Boundaries," in *Loving Bravely: 20 Lessons of Self-Discovery to Help You Get the Love You Want* (Oakland, CA: New Harbinger Publications, 2017), 48.

11. Making It Stick

256 **us as adults:** Mona DeKoven Fishbane, "Healing Intergenerational Wounds: An Integrative Relational–Neurobiological Approach," *Family Process* 58, no. 4 (2019): 796–818, doi: 10.1111/famp.12488.

256 **daily physical exercise:** John J. Ratey with Eric Hagerman, *Spark: The Revolutionary New Science of Exercise and the Brain* (New York: Little, Brown Spark, 2008).

256 **and pay attention:** Norman Doidge, "Redesigning the Brain," in *The Brain That Changes Itself: Stories of Personal Triumph from the Frontiers of Brain Science* (London: Penguin Books, 2008), 45–92.

257   **in unhappy relationships:** Janice K. Kiecolt-Glaser and Ronald Glaser, "Psychological Stress, Telomeres, and Telomerase," *Brain, Behavior, and Immunity* 24, no. 4 (2010): 529–30, doi: 10.1016/j.bbi.2010.02.002.

257   **healthiest at age eighty:** Robert Waldinger, "What Makes a Good Life? Lessons from the Longest Study on Happiness," filmed November 2015 at TEDxBeaconStreet, Brookline, MA, video, 12:38, https://youtu.be/8KkKuTCFvzI.

258   **"not push love away":** Melanie Curtin, "This 75-Year Harvard Study Found the 1 Secret to Leading a Fulfilling Life," *Grow* (blog), *Inc.*, February 27, 2017, https://www.inc.com/melanie-curtin/want-a-life-of-fulfillment-a-75 -year-harvard-study-says-to-prioritize-this-one-t.html.

Conclusion

269   **systems you're in:** Harriet Goldhor Lerner, *The Dance of Anger: A Woman's Guide to Changing the Patterns of Intimate Relationships* (New York: HarperCollins, 1985).

271   **parents as real people:** James L. Framo, "The Integration of Marital Therapy with Sessions with Family of Origin," in *Handbook of Family Therapy*, ed. Alan S. Gurman and David P. Kniskern (New York: Brunner/Mazel, 1981), 133–57.

271   **Michael Kerr:** Mona DeKoven Fishbane, "Healing Intergenerational Wounds: An Integrative Relational-Neurobiological Approach," *Family Process* 58, no. 4 (2019): 796–818, doi:10.111/famp.12488.

INDEX

abandonment
    feeling worthy and, 64 (*see also*
        worthiness wound)
    threats of, 160–61 (*see also* safety
        wound)
    trust and, 141–43, 149
abuse, 158–62
accountability, 193
adaptation, 99–100
addiction examples, 162, 228
adults. *See* parental figures
advice, giving vs. receiving, 48
aggressive communication, 213,
    220–23
Ainsworth, Mary, 147
All About Love (hooks), 158
Angelou, Maya, 99
anxious attachment, 147–50
attachment
    Attachment Theory, 147–50
    authenticity vs., 25–27, 259–62
authenticity
    attachment vs., 25–27, 259–62
    belonging and, 85, 103–4 (*see also*
        belonging wound)
    healing for authentic love, 258
    inauthentic connection, 241–44
    leading with, for healing, 259–62
avoidance

belonging and, 89–91
naming your wound and, 42
trusting and, 152–54
awareness
    of communication style, 233
    of fear, 219
    for identifying wound, 37–40,
        208–9 (*see also* wounds and their
        origins)
    pausing for, 262–64
    relational self-awareness, 210–11
    of roles in family of origin, 22–25
    as worthwhile process, 258
    of your own shortcomings, 269–71

behavior of others
    relating to, 11
    repeating dysfunctional patterns,
        44, 46–47
belonging wound, 85–108
    accommodating others and
        effect on, 26
    communication and, 232–33
    conflict and, 196–97
    control, 91–93
    coping with, 99–104
    healing of, 104–6
    ignoring and avoidance, 89–91
    intolerance and shame, 93–95

belonging wound (*cont.*)
   naming wounds of, 38
   Origin Healing Practice for, 106–8
   origins of, overview, 85–89
   societal impact, 95–99
   writing prompts for, 91, 93, 95,
      98–99, 105
betrayal, 22–25, 39, 135–36, 137–39.
   See also trust wound
biracial identity, 96–98
birth story secrets, 140–41
blended families. *See* stepfamilies
body image examples, 70–72, 101–2
The Body Keeps the Score (Van Der
   Kolk), 165
boundaries, 236–52
   courageous acts and, 246–49
   creating, 74
   healthy boundaries blocked by
      wounds, 240–41
   healthy vs. unhealthy, overview,
      236–38
   inauthentic connection as block to,
      241–44
   porous, 238–39, 244–46, 251
   questions about (exercises), 245,
      247–48
   rigid, 239–40, 249–52
   writing prompts about, 241, 248
Bowlby, John, 147
Brown, Brené, 19, 104, 131

caretakers. *See* parental figures
changing relationship behaviors,
   183–252
   boundaries and, 236–52
      (*see also* boundaries)
   communication and, 210–35
      (*see also* communication)
   conflict and, 185–209
      (*see also* conflict)
   inability to change, 194–95
   making it stick, 255–67
      (*see also* healing)
character, attack on, 190–92

children, exploitation of, 162
children, wounds of. *See* family
   of origin; wounds and their
   origins
closing off, 143–44
code-switching, 96–98
communication, 210–35. *See also*
   boundaries
   aggressive, 213, 220–23
   as choice, 212–13
   clarity of, 232–34
   disorganized, 213, 227–32
   for freedom, 234–25
   identifying style of, 233
   inauthentic connection as block to,
      241–44
   passive, 213–20
   passive-aggressive, 213, 223–27
   unblocking, overview, 213
   for understanding, 210–11
   writing prompts about, 217,
      218, 219
conditional love, 67–69
conditioning, 22–25
conflict, 185–209. *See also* boundaries;
   communication
   being seen, heard, and understood,
      187–88
   as connection attempt, 186
   constructive, 186
   contemptuousness and, 199–203
   control and, 196–99
   criticism and, 189–92
   defensiveness and, 192–95
   examining, 185
   identifying wound and, 37–40,
      208–9
   origins of, 188–89
   stonewalling and, 203–5
   understanding vs. reactivity for,
      205–8
   writing prompts about, 207–8
connection
   conflict as attempt for, 186, 199
   healing for, 258

inauthentic, as block to
communication/boundaries,
241–44
with yourself and others, 213,
223–27 (*see also* communication)
constraint, understanding, 218
constraint question, 40
contemptuousness, 199–203
control. *See also* safety wound
belonging and, 91–93
conflict and, 196–99
as protection, 226
"counting to ten," 262–64
couples therapy, needs of, 110
courageous acts, 246–49
covert expectations, 113
criticism, 189–92
cultural abuse, 161

"Dear Trust Wound" letter
(exercise), 156
deceit, 136, 140–41
defensiveness, 192–95
discernment, 150, 152, 212, 218
disorganized communication, 213,
227–32
dissociation, 165–67
distraction (of family of origin),
116–18
domesticshelters.org, 158
dysfunction, intergenerational, 12
dysfunctional patterns, repeating,
44, 46–47

economic abuse, 161
emergency hotlines, 158
emotion
emotional abuse, 160
Emotionally Focused Therapy, 196
emotional needs, 205–8
emotional tending, 202
emotional wounds, 37–38 (*see also*
naming your wound)
understanding vs. reactivity, 205–8,
210–11

Epston, David, 130–31
estrangement, 7
exercises
for belonging wound, 91, 93, 95,
98–99, 105
for boundaries, 241, 245, 247–48
for communication, 217, 218, 219
journaling for, 35
for safety wound, 165, 167, 169,
180–82
for trust wound, 139, 141, 142–43,
153, 156
for worthiness wound, 57–58, 66,
71, 73, 83
expectations
covert, 113
family rules and, 91–93
of safety, 157–58 (*see also* safety
wound)
exploitation of children, 162

factual storytelling, 61–62
family of origin
defined, 32–33
intergenerational dysfunction
and, 12
multiple families of origin, 33–34
naming your wound and, 31–53
(*see also* naming your wound)
parental figures, defined, 9
preoccupation and distraction of,
116–118
repeating dysfunctional patterns
of, 44, 46–47
safety wound occurring with, 1–5
(*see also* safety wound)
your past experiences with, 17–30
(*see also* past as present)
Far from the Tree (Solomon), 90
fear
fear of missing out (FOMO), 96
identifying, 219
living in, 169–73
of "other shoe dropping," 18, 19, 24
scary situations and safety, 167–69

financial abuse, 161
financial behavior example, 163–64
FOMO (fear of missing out), 96
"The Four Horsemen of the
    Apocalypse," 189
Frankl, Viktor, 262, 264
freedom, communication as, 234–35

"geographical cure," 7
Glover, Robert, 113
Gottman, John, 189, 205–8
grieving loss step, 75, 78–79, 82–83.
    See also Origin Healing Practice
groundedness in communication,
    213, 227–32

harm, statements of, 69–72
Harvard University, 257–58
healing. *See also* changing
    relationship behaviors;
    exercises
  change as realistic, 256–58
  integration for, 255–56, 258
  leading with authenticity for,
    259–62
  for peace vs. suffering, 264–65
  respecting pause for, 262–64
  as sacred experience, 81
  self-love and, 266–67
  as work in progress, 267
healthy boundaries. *See* boundaries
Hemingway, Ernest, 151
hiding, 41
honor others (for communication),
    213, 220–23
honor your voice (for
    communication), 213–20
hooks, bell, 158
horizontals, 90
hypervigilance, 144–45

identity, racial/biracial/multiracial,
    96–98
identity abuse, 161
ignoring, 89–91
"I'll do it if . . ." game, 216–17

inconsistency, 64–65
Instagram, 6
integration, 255–56, 258
Integrative Systemic Therapy, 7
intergenerational transmission of
    psychopathology, 121
intimacy, healing for, 258.
    See also healing
intolerance, 93–95
"The Invitation Day" (Oriah), 236

Johnson, Susan, 196
journaling, 35
Jung, Carl, 63

Kerr, Michael, 271

LGBT example, 85–89, 93–94
Loving Bravely (Solomon), 238

Maté, Gabor, 26, 180
mental abuse, 160–61
mental health example, 175–78
Messi, Lionel, 257
mindfulness, 180–82
multiracial identity, 96–98

naming your wound, 31–53
  concealing wounds, cost of, 43–48
  family of origin as source of
    wound, 32–34 (*see also* family
    of origin)
  importance of, 31–32, 52–53
  naming wound step (Origin
    Healing Practice), 75–76, 81–82
    (*see also* Origin Healing
    Practice)
  process of, 49–52
  relational dynamics in families
    and, 34–36
  revealing wound for, 37–40, 208–9
narrative therapy, 130–31
National Domestic Violence
    Hotline, 158
neglect, 161–62
No More Mr. Nice Guy! (Glover), 113

opposition, 123–26, 255
Oriah, 236
Origin Healing Practice, 75–84
   for belonging wound, 106–8
   grieving loss, 75, 78–79, 82–83
   guided meditation for safety
      wound, 180–82
   healing as sacred experience for, 81
   naming wound, 75–76, 81–82
   pivoting to new behaviors, 75,
      79–80, 83–84
   for prioritization wound, 132–34
   witnessing wound, 75, 76–78, 82
origin healing work
   origin story as story of firsts, 34
   overview, 6, 10–13
   revealing wound for, 37–38
      (see also naming your wound)
origin of you, 1–13. See also family of
   origin; origin healing work;
   safety wound
   origin healing work and, 6, 10–13
   recognizing safety wound, 5–10
   safety wound occurring with
      family of origin, 1–5
origin relational wounding, 131–32
origin stories. See family of origin
origin wound, 6
others, awareness of pain to, 269–71
ownership, avoiding, 193

parental figures
   defined, 9
   harmful messaging by, 25–27
   intergenerational transmission of
      psychopathology, 121
   parents' unresolved wounds, 118–20
   relational dynamics with, 34–36
   repeating patterns of, 44
passive-aggressive communication,
   213, 223–27
passive communication, 213–20
past as present, 17–30
   acknowledging past experiences,
      17–22, 28–30
   authenticity vs. attachment, 25–27

recognizing your role in family of
   origin, 22–25
pause, respecting, 262–64
peace vs. suffering, 264–65
people-pleasing behavior, 4, 43, 239,
   244. See also boundaries
performing, 42
perspective (blowing things out of
   proportion), 45–46
Pharaon, Vienna. See also Origin
   Healing Practice
   Instagram community of, 6
   personal story of, 1–5, 40, 67–69,
      77–78, 144–45, 236–37, 246–49
physical abuse, 159
physical disability example, 89–91
pivoting to new behaviors
   for change, 198–99 (see also
      changing relationship behaviors)
   Origin Healing Practice step, 75,
      79–80, 83–84
pleasing, 42–43
porous boundaries, 238–39,
   244–46, 251
Poston, Walker S. Carlos, 97
power. See control
"The Power of Vulnerability"
   (Brown), 19
preoccupation (of family of origin),
   116–18
presenting problem, 6
prioritization wound, 109–34
   accommodating others and
      effect on, 26
   communication and, 227–32
   conflict and, 196–97
   coping with, 120–26
   healing of, 126–32
   naming wounds of, 38
   Origin Healing Practice for, 132–34
   origins of, overview, 110–16
   parents' unresolved wounds, 118–20
   preoccupied/distracted family of
      origin, 116–18
   prioritization, defined, 109–10
   recognizing patterns of, 11

professional help, seeking, 158.
  See also therapy
protection, 22, 226
psychological abuse, 160–61

racial abuse, 161
racial identity, 96–98
reactivity
  naming wound and, 44–45
  understanding vs., 205–8, 210–11
Real, Terry, 12
reassurance, 68
rebuilding of trust, 150–54
recklessness, 162–65
reclamation, making change stick,
  255–67. *See also* healing
rejection, 101–3
relational dynamics, 34–36.
  See also changing relationship
  behaviors
relational self-awareness, 210–11
religion examples, 94–95, 161
repetition, 121–23, 255
Rhimes, Shonda, 234–35
rigid boundaries, 239–40, 249–52
Rising Strong (Brown), 131
roles (in family of origin), 22–25
romantic relationships
  fertility issues example, 49–52
  recognizing patterns in, 11
  secrets example, 22–25, 39
rules, 91–93

sabotage, 47–48, 145–47
safety wound, 157–82.
  See also naming your wound
  abuse, 158–62
  accommodating others and
    effect on, 26
  communication and, 227–33
  conflict and, 195
  control and, 92
  coping with, 169–78
  dissociation, 165–67
  expectations of safety, 157–58
  healing of, 178–80

naming wounds of, 38
occurring with family of origin, 1–5
Origin Healing Practice for
  (guided meditation), 180–82
origins of, overview, 158
origin wound, 6
recklessness, 162–65
  recognizing, 5–10
  scary situations, 167–69
  writing prompts about, 165, 167, 169
scary situations, 167–69
Schnarch, David, 102
secrets, burden of, 22–25, 39, 135–36,
  137–39
seen, feeling, 187–88. *See also* conflict;
  witnessing wound
self-awareness, relational, 210–11
self-love, 266–67
sexual abuse, 159–60
shame, 93–95
shapeshifting, accommodating others
  as, 4, 27, 260
shutting down, 173–78
societal impact, 95–99
Solomon, Alexandra, 12, 179,
  210–11, 238
Solomon, Andrew, 90
statements of harm, 69–72
stepfamilies
  as multiple families of origin,
    33–34
  trust in, 137–39, 145–47
stonewalling, 203–5, 240
storytelling, factual, 61–62
Strange Situation study, 147–50
suffering, peace vs., 264–65

Tawwab, Nedra Glover, 238
TEDx talk, "The Power of
  Vulnerability" (Brown), 19
testing, 145–47
therapy
  constraint question in, 40
  for couples, 110
  Emotionally Focused Therapy, 196
  Integrative Systemic Therapy, 7

making progress in, 229–30
naming your wound for
 effectiveness of, 31–32
 (*see also* naming your wound)
narrative, 130–31
origin healing work, 6, 10–13
 (*see also* origin healing work)
presenting problem, 6
recognizing patterns in your past
 for, 17–22
trauma. *See* safety wound; trust
 wound; wounds and their
 origins
trust wound, 135–56
 abandonment and, 141–43
 accommodating others and
  effect on, 26
 betrayal and, 135–36, 137–39
 betrayal and burden of secrets,
  22–25, 39
 coping with, 143–50
 "Dear Trust Wound" letter
  (exercise), 156
 deceit and, 136, 140–41
 healing of, 150–54
 naming wounds of, 38, 39–40
 Origin Healing Practice for, 154–56
 origins of, overview, 136–37
 recognizing patterns of, 11
 stonewalling and, 203–5, 240
 trauma and trust, 179–80
 writing prompts for, 139, 141,
  142–43, 153
truth, recognizing, 11

unavailability, 63–66
understanding
 feeling understood, 187–88
  (*see also* conflict)
 reactivity vs., 205–8, 210–11

unhealthy boundaries.
 See boundaries

Vaillant, George, 257–58
Van Der Kolk, Bessel, 165
Vanzant, Iyanla, 80
verbal abuse, 160
vulnerability, 43, 173–78.
 See also naming your wound

Walsh, Froma, 7
White, Michael, 130–31
witnessing wound, 75, 76–78, 82
worthiness wound, 57–74
 accommodating others and
  effect on, 26
 boundaries and, 247
 communication and, 225–26, 233
 conditional love and, 67–69
 coping with, 72–73
 examples of feeling unworthy,
  59–63
 naming wounds of, 38
 overview, 57–59
 statements of harm and,
  69–72
 unavailability and, 63–66
 writing prompts for, 57–58, 66, 71,
  73, 83
wounds and their origins, 55–182.
 See also changing relationship
  behaviors
 identifying wound, 37–40, 208–9
  (*see also* naming your wound)
 Origin Healing Practice for,
  75–84 (*see also* Origin Healing
  Practice)
 worthiness, 57–74 (*see also*
  worthiness wound)
writing prompts. *See* exercises